Evaluating Clinical Change

Strategies for Occupational and Physical Therapists

Evaluating Clinical Change

Strategies for Occupational and Physical Therapists

KENNETH J. OTTENBACHER
Ph.D., O.T.R.

Assistant Professor
University of Wisconsin-Madison
School of Allied Health Professions
Madison, Wisconsin

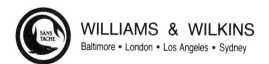

WILLIAMS & WILKINS
Baltimore • London • Los Angeles • Sydney

Editor: John P. Butler
Associate Editor: Victoria Vaughn
Copy Editor: Bill Cady
Design: JoAnne Janowiak
Illustration Planning: Reginald R. Stanley
Production: Raymond E. Reter

Printed in the United States of America

Library of Congress Cataloging in Publication Data
Ottenbacher, Kenneth J.
  Evaluating clinical change.

  Bibliography: p.
  Includes index.
  1. Occupational therapy—Evaluation. 2. Physical therapy—Evaluation. 3. Occupational therapy—Research. 4. Physical therapy—Research. I. Title.
[DNLM: 1. Evaluation Studies. 2. Occupational Therapy. 3. Physical Therapy.
4. Research Design. WB 460 089e]
RM735.088 1986   615.8′515   85-9247
ISBN 0-683-06659-5

88 89   10 9 8 7 6 5 4 3

To Margaret and my daughters who . . .

The purpose of evaluation is to improve, not to prove.
DANIEL L. STUFFLEBEAM

Preface

The need for systematic scientific inquiry in occupational and physical therapy has been widely documented during the past decade. Numerous authors have repeatedly identified the professional risks associated with a failure to establish a scientific data base to validate clinical practice. Indeed, some authorities (Basmajian, 1975) have questioned the continued viability of specific rehabilitation specialties if this empirical foundation is not developed. Obviously, the disciplines of occupational and physical therapy have chosen to pursue professional status within the rehabilitation service hierarchy and are vigorously encouraging research as an integral aspect of professional development. The number of data-based empirical investigations reported in the occupational and physical therapy literature has increased dramatically over the past five or six years.

The underlying premise of this text is that we need to emphasize not only the production of research but also the integration of empirical findings and methods into clinical practice. There is a definite distinction in the health related professions between research production and research utilization (Fuhrer, 1983). The purpose of this text is to promote the use of systematic research and evaluation strategies in clinical practice. Unfortunately, many therapists are not employing the available principles of scientific inquiry in their clinical practice. The failure to establish a nexus between research and clinical practice may ultimately negate many of the recent advances that we have made in terms of research production. As Christiansen (1983, p. 197) recently observed, "our greatest challenge is to overcome the attitude of neglect toward scientific inquiry. Unfortunately, research continues to be viewed commonly as an activity foreign to our clinics and irrelevant to our practice."

One goal of this text is to demonstrate to therapists that certain types of evaluation and research activities can be conducted in clinical settings and are relevant to clinical practice. In fact, with the increased emphasis on therapeutic accountability, DRGs, etc., properly conducted evaluation and research will certainly be an essential part of clinical practice in the decades to come.

The argument will be made throughout the first three chapters that traditional group-comparison research, with its emphasis on large samples, between-group comparisons, and sophisticated statistical inference, is often of limited relevance to the practicing therapist. The therapist working in a clinical setting is generally concerned with documenting client progress on an individual basis.

Traditional "experimental" designs are well established in the scientific community and are capable of verifying theoretically derived predictions (hypotheses). The primary function of traditional between-group designs is to validate theories used in clinical practice. If a theory is supported by traditional large-N group-comparison research, the theory can serve as a legitimate guide for clinical practice. Group designs based on large-N methodology, however, are often of limited use in documenting the clinical progress of an individual client or patient receiving therapy services. The decision rules and tenets of statistical inference associated with traditional between-group designs are based on comparisons of average performance across groups and provide little information related to the behavior of an individual patient.

The information presented throughout this text details procedures based on single system evaluation and research strategies that are designed to assess individual client performance in a clinical environment. These procedures provide the therapist with a systematic and objective mechanism of documenting clinical change over time. The procedures can be implemented in any setting and are recognized as scientifically valid and empirically respected methods for conducting clinical research.

The material covered in the text is sometimes complex, and my efforts to present the information in a clear and scholarly manner may occasionally fail. Therapeutically relevant examples have been included whenever possible in an attempt to minimize these didactic failures. Numerous graphs and figures have also been included to assist those individuals who, like myself, learn more easily from "pictures" than from words. Finally, I hope that I have not distorted or misrepresented the material presented. As to errors in scholarship, quotes, conceptualization, and syntax, may my friends and colleagues correct me—quietly.

References

Basmajian, J. V. (1975). Research or retrench: The rehabilitation professions challenged. *Phys. Ther., 55,* 607–610.

Christiansen, C. H. (1983). Editorial—Research: An economic imperative. *Occup. Ther. J. Res., 3,* 195–198.

Fuhrer, M. J. (1983). Communicating and utilizing research in medical rehabilitation. *Arch. Phys. Med. Rehabil., 64,* 608–610.

Acknowledgments

Rarely is an author able to create truly original material or generate new information and insights. Most authors, myself included, must be satisfied with synthesizing and rearranging existing information. The ideas, procedures, and concepts contained in this book are not original. They were developed and refined by numerous teachers, clinicians, and researchers to whom I owe a debut of intellectual gratitude. I have attempted to place their ideas in a context that will make the information relevant to occupational and physical therapists.

I am grateful to Peg Short-Degraff, Paul Petersen, Jennifer Angelo, and Alice Punwar who read earlier drafts of the material presented in the text and provided valuable suggestions and encouragement. Finally, I owe a large thank you to Ann Rhoads who demonstrated inexhaustible patience along with superior word processing ability in producing several drafts of the text.

K. J. O.

Contents

Preface ix

Acknowledgments xi

CHAPTER 1_____
Evaluating Clinical Change: Implications for Research and
Practice. 1

CHAPTER 2_____
Traditional Research Methods: The Group-Comparison
Approach. 21

CHAPTER 3_____
Introduction to Single System Evaluation Strategies. 43

CHAPTER 4_____
Measurement and Recording Procedures Associated with Single
System Designs 65

CHAPTER 5_____
Basic Designs for Single System Evaluation and Research . . 89

CHAPTER 6_____
Intermediate and Advanced Designs for Single System Evaluation
and Research 111

CHAPTER 7
Visual Analysis of Single System Data **137**

CHAPTER 8
Statistical Analysis of Single System Data **167**

CHAPTER 9
Single System Strategies: Summing Up **197**

Glossary **217**

References **227**

Index **237**

CHAPTER 1

Evaluating Clinical Change: Implications for Research and Practice

RESEARCH IN OCCUPATIONAL AND PHYSICAL THERAPY: AN OVERVIEW

During the past 10 to 15 years, there has been a concerted effort in both occupational and physical therapy to establish a scientific foundation for clinical practice and to develop a research literature unique to the respective disciplines. This effort has resulted in a dramatic increase in the number of research reports appearing in the professional literature. For example, Ottenbacher and Short (1982) recently reviewed publication trends in the *American Journal of Occupational Therapy* for the period 1970 to 1980. They classified all the articles appearing during that decade into one of seven categories. The seven categories included articles labeled as descriptive, survey, case and field studies, correlational, quasi-experimental, true experimental and practical. Data analysis revealed that a significant change in the type of articles appearing in the *Journal* had occurred during the decade. Specifically, there was an increase in data-based articles labeled as quasi-experimental in which an independent and dependent variable were clearly identified and a test of a hypothesis was conducted. Conversely,

1

there was a corresponding decrease in the number of articles labeled as descriptive (see Figure 1.1). Descriptive articles included those reports in which a particular treatment program, theory, or area of practice was discussed. Historical and review articles were also included in this category.

The analysis by Ottenbacher and Short (1982) provides quantitative evidence that therapists are realizing they can no longer be complacent

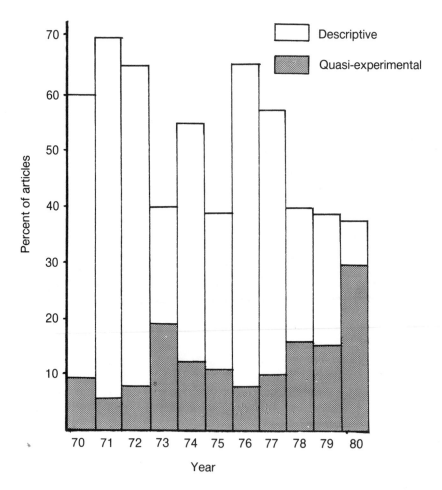

Figure 1.1. Comparison of quasi-experimental and descriptive articles published between 1970 and 1980 in the *American Journal of Occupational Therapy.* (Adapted from: Ottenbacher, K., and Short, M. A. (1982). Publication trends in occupational therapy. *Occup. Ther. J. Res., 2,* 80–88.)

regarding the scientific justification of the therapeutic interventions they employ. A cursory review of many of the currently popular treatment procedures and modalities employed by therapists reveals that the research supporting many of them is not as strong as the ''faith'' in them. Providing adequate empirical evidence for the effectiveness of currently employed intervention strategies will provide a major challenge for occupational and physical therapy researchers and clinicians throughout the 1980s. Indeed, several authorities in the field of rehabilitation have argued, persuasively, that a credible research base for practice will be the *raison d'être* of both physical and occupational therapy in the near future (Christiansen, 1981; Hislop, 1975). A failure to establish and support a strong research foundation will constitute a tacit admission by members of the rehabilitation-related disciplines that they are satisfied with a technical role in providing health care services.

In a provocative article written several years ago entitled, ''Research or Retrench: The Rehabilitation Professions Challenged,'' Basmajian (1975) argued that the rehabilitation disciplines, including occupational and physical therapy, were at a crossroads in terms of professional development. He observed that members of the rehabilitation specialties could actively pursue a professional status within the rehabilitation services hierarchy by encouraging research and scholarly activity in their respective fields or, alternatively, they could allow the disciplines to continue on their present (1975) course and become ''respected technologies.'' Basmajian (1975) emphasized that members of each discipline had the opportunity to make a collective choice. He also noted that by not actively pursuing professionalization through research, members of these disciplines would be passively accepting for their discipline the role of ''respected technology.'' In a subsequent article, Basmajian (1977) noted that if the decision were made to move toward an independent professional status, a fundamental change in attitude would be required in the education and training of rehabilitation ''professionals.'' Specifically, Basmajian (1977) argued that professionals in the fields of physical and occupational therapy must concentrate less on teaching technique and de-emphasize the ''how to'' nature of their curriculums and become more concerned with ''why'' questions, exploring the theory and rationale behind the procedures that are taught and advocated as therapeutically effective.

Many changes have occurred since Basmajian wrote these articles. Members of the disciplines of occupational and physical therapy have obviously chosen to pursue professional status and are vigorously promoting and encouraging members to contribute to the research literature in the respective fields. Physical therapists are in the process of enacting a mandate to raise the entry level to a postbaccalaureate degree. This mandate is obviously designed, in part, to enhance the academic and scholarly skills of entry level practitioners so that they will become more sophisticated consumers and producers of research literature.

The movement toward establishing the empirical legitimacy of many therapeutic procedures employed by occupational and physical therapists is in its infancy and will continue for many years before definitive decisions can be made regarding the efficacy of particular intervention strategies. In the meantime, therapeutic programs are being developed and provided to individual patients or groups of clients on a regular basis. Methods and procedures to evaluate the therapeutic usefulness of the programs as currently applied to *specific individuals* are urgently needed. The purpose of this text is to provide practitioners with a set of guidelines and procedures to evaluate clinical change in patients. These procedures are similar in some cases to those employed in applied research studies. The goal of these procedures, however, is generally conceived as more circumspect than that associated with traditional research. The procedures are employed specifically to measure clinical change, usually on an individual or small group basis. The primary goal is not to evaluate theoretical hypotheses or to test theoretical predictions. In addition, there is little attempt to generalize the findings of the evaluation methodology beyond the individual clients or the situations that are clinically relevant. The findings of such evaluation research may have secondary implications for theory development or refinement; the primary purpose of this research, however, is to demonstrate the efficacy of *in situ* applications of a therapeutic procedure.

The demonstration of clinical effectiveness should be an integral part of any structured therapeutic program carried out in physical or occupational therapy clinics. In the current economic and political climate, no health care professional can hope to defend his or her discipline against skepticism and accusations of inefficiency or questionable ethical integrity unless its treatment programs demonstrate therapeutic results. For instance, Gillette (1982, p. 499) recently observed that "the practice claims of the profession must be established in order to provide ample evidence of the value of occupational therapy to consumers of the service and to other health care providers as well. In the absence of careful and thorough documentation, members of a profession such as occupational therapy will not receive appropriate recognition nor adequate reimbursement for their services."

Along similar lines, Payton (1979, p. IX) states, "Research is important to therapy because it is the major tool available to us for validating our services to people in our roles as therapists." The general validity of therapeutic procedures is gradually established over a period of time via the accumulation of research evidence supporting or refuting a particular theoretical position. Such validation of particular therapeutic programs applied to special handicapping conditions or populations is essential to the professional development of physical and occupational therapy, but it is not the only form of therapeutic validity. As clinicians we must also be able to demonstrate the ''validity'' of the specific therapeutic procedures applied to *individual* clients in *specific clinical environments*. We must be concerned with the ''individual'' validity of our therapeutic procedures as well as their theoretical validity. The procedures presented in this text are designed to evaluate specific changes in client behavior or performance on an individual or small group basis. They are not designed or intended to provide information that will directly facilitate theory development, and they are not meant to be inferential or generalizable in the usual empirical sense associated with traditional research paradigms that rely on comparisons of performance between a treatment and a control group. The goal with use of these procedures is to provide a mechanism or methodology for evaluating clinical change on a case-by-case basis. Such a goal is conceptualized as inherently continuous in nature. It is the obligation of all therapists to provide consumers of their services with systematic information related to the effectiveness of the services provided. The application of small-N designs and related procedures described in subsequent chapters of this text will assist therapists in meeting this professional obligation in a systematic, objective manner. Yet the single system methods described cannot be the sole type of research relevant to practice. The clinical value of single system evaluation strategies can be realized best in relation to more traditional methods that emphasize group-comparison designs. An understanding of the strengths and weaknesses of both single system and group-comparison designs is necessary to appreciate the relative merits of each approach in the establishment of a clinical research base that can influence practice. Information necessary to place traditional group-comparison designs and single system strategies in the broader context of clinical evaluation and research is presented in Chapters 2 and 3.

The selection of programs and techniques of therapeutic intervention for a particular handicapped population or handicapping condition must be based on clear empirical evidence of effectiveness. This clear empirical evidence regarding the overall effectiveness of a treatment program generally requires the use of traditional group-comparison (large-N) research designs. For the most part, this is because of difficulties in generalizing to target populations or multiple clinical settings with use of small-N or single system designs. One of the major advantages of traditional group-comparison research procedures in which large numbers of randomly selected and assigned subjects are employed is precisely that rules for generalizing evidence are well defined.

It can be argued that not every occupational or physical therapy clinic should, or even could, be involved in the production of traditional large-N group-comparison research to test hypotheses or develop and refine theory related to therapeutic practice. Every clinical therapist providing service, however, has the responsibility to document, in a systematic manner, the effectiveness or noneffectiveness of the service provided to any given client. The purpose of this text is to make available to students and practitioners in occupational and physical therapy the knowledge, skills, and specific procedures to evaluate their own practices. The primary tool advocated for achieving this goal is the small-N or "intensive" design. These procedures, also referred to as single subject designs, single-case experimental designs, time-series designs or idiographic research, are systematic ways of analyzing, measuring, and evaluating practice. Although single subject designs were originally developed for studying a single individual, they are, in fact, quite applicable to treatment evaluation in two ways: (1) the replication of several single subject designs applied to individuals; and (2) the substitution of small groups of subjects or program criteria for the individual subject. These two applications make the term single *system* designs more appropriate for the strategies presented in this text. The first approach may involve the use of multiple single system designs in order to determine intervention effects across several clients, settings, or types of disorders. This approach is based on the way investigators have traditionally conducted single-case experiments. On the other hand, the second approach would be based on treatment outcome measures or measurements gathered on a small group of clients as the outcome variable. Each data point may represent either a specific program outcome measure or an "average" across a small number of subjects.

Regardless of whether single system designs are used to study the effects of programs or treatments on individuals or small groups, two major aspects of single system procedures are stressed: (1) the sequential or varied application and/or withdrawal of the intervention; and (2) the use of frequent and repeated outcome measures. The variety and the complexity of single system design options available to therapists have increased dramatically in the past decade, as is evident in later chapters. Even the most sophisticated and complex single system designs, however, retain the basic features described previously. Small-N evaluation research involves approaches and procedures that demonstrate how clinical practice and applied research can be integrated, which thus offers an excellent opportunity for clinicians to demonstrate their accountability and to validate their intervention strategies simultaneously. Moreover, as is discussed in later chapters, single system evaluation research methods have a number of specific advantages that allow these methods to be easily adapted to practice environments.

Prior to a detailed discussion of the specific procedures and methodology recommended for evaluating individual clinical change, a brief review of the relationship of traditional research and theory to clinical practice is provided. It is hoped that this introductory material will begin to highlight the similarities and differences between traditional group-comparison methods and the single system strategies that are presented in later chapters.

Research, Theory and Practice

Until recently, the primary professional concern relating to research in occupational and physical therapy centered around the need to accomplish this research. The emphasis on the production of data-based research included encouraging qualified therapists to conduct research and providing them with the necessary funding and support services. Many of the professional associations' resources were channeled toward the goal of research production. This goal is now being realized. As reported previously, there has been a noticeable increase in the number of data-based research reports appearing in the therapy literature over the past decade (Ottenbacher and Short, 1982). Now that a research literature is emerging and methods of disseminating research findings have been developed (Llorens, 1981), a shift in emphasis is indicated. More emphasis should now be devoted toward integrating and utilizing occupational and physical therapy research in clinical practice.

All professionals and members of those disciplines for which professional status is sought make the assumption that research will somehow have an impact on professional practice (Goode, 1969). For example, several leaders in nursing have argued, more by exhortation than evidence, that nursing research is important practically and is having an impact on patient care (Gortner, 1975; Gortner and Nahm, 1977). This declaration can be found in most applied disciplines. Certainly, more research is being conducted in health-related fields, including occupational and physical therapy, now than in the past. The question is, to what extent is that research having an impact on clinical practice?

A study in nursing practice illustrates the nature of the problem. Ketefian (1975) investigated the extent to which a specific research finding which was related to the recording of oral body temperature was used by practicing nurses. The finding, documented through a series of studies and widely disseminated over a period of 5 years, had obvious applications to nursing practice. Nevertheless, based on her survey, Ketefian (1973, p. 91) concluded that "the practitioner either was totally unaware of the research literature relative to her practice, or if she was aware of it, was unable to relate to it or utilize it."

The problem illustrated in this study of nursing practice is certainly germane to occupational and physical therapy. The accumulating evidence suggests that much applied research based on traditional group-comparison models and designed to be relevant for professional practice in applied fields is seldom utilized (Barlow et al., 1984; Ballin et al., 1980; Hunt, 1981; Strupp, 1981). In discussing the attitude of occupational therapists toward research utilization, Christiansen (1983, p. 197) recently observed, "Our greatest challenge is to overcome the attitude of neglect toward scientific inquiry. Unfortunately, research continues to be viewed commonly as an activity foreign to our clinics and irrelevant to our practice." The argument is made throughout this text that treatment evaluation strategies designed for use with individual clients can help bridge the research-practice gap.

The purpose of research in occupational and physical therapy is to enhance the knowledge base related to practice, so that consumers receive the best available treatment. It is axiomatic, therefore, that both producers of research and direct service providers should be concerned with the effectiveness with which information generated through research and evaluation is incorporated into practice. As Fuhrer (1983, p. 610) recently observed, "the provision of rehabilitation services that are grounded in systematic research is something owed to the persons we serve and something required if our practice is to be viewed as credible by the informed public. However, mere availability of more and better research will not assure incorporation of knowledge into practice."

For a full appreciation of the complex process of research utilization, it is necessary to develop a broad understanding of research and evaluation activities and the relationship of research and evaluation methods to clinical practice. One obvious method of applying research results to practice situations is to extrapolate the findings from a single study and apply them directly to the clinical setting. This approach may have a certain degree of direct intuitive appeal, but it is not the most desirable method of synthesizing research and practice. Burr et al. (1973) refer to this approach as the "empirical method." They go on to explain that the direct application of results from a specific study to a particular clinical setting has some serious limitations in the production of useful therapeutic outcomes. The "empirical method" is likely to be limited by the absence of an exact fit between client problems and those reported in the investigation. A second limitation is the clinician's general inability to replicate the precise intervention strategies employed by the original investigators. This limitation may be related to the failure of the researcher to provide enough operational detail concerning the treatment, or it may be a function of the therapist's particular setting or circumstance. The therapist, for instance, may not have the proper piece of equipment or necessary space or resources to carry out the intervention as originally described by the investigator. For instance, Chee et al. (1978) conducted a study in which children with cerebral palsy were subjected to a program of controlled vestibular stimulation. The stimulation was provided in a darkened room while the child was positioned in a specially adapted rotating chair. The program required a ratio of 2 adults to 1 child. The results of the investigation indicated that the patients receiving the vestibular stimulation displayed a significant degree of improvement on measures of reflex integration and gross motor skills. A clinical therapist reading this report might be tempted to adapt the general procedures employed by Chee et al. (i.e., the use of rotatory vestibular stimulation) and might expect to produce the same results reported by the original investigators. It is doubtful, however, that the clinical therapist would be able to replicate the procedures that Chee et al. used. In most clinical settings the staff, space or equipment to adequately or accurately replicate this study is not available. The therapist's assumption that adapting the procedures used by Chee et al. would produce the same results in his or her own clinical setting is not valid and represents a misinterpretation of clinical research based on traditional experimental group-comparison methods.

Williamson (1982) has also observed that the results of any given study may be unique to the sample employed or to some interaction of sample characteristics and research design. The variability associated with isolated research findings, particularly in much rehabilitation research where populations and samples often consist of individuals with disorders or dysfunctions that make them very heterogeneous, makes the direct application of the findings to a clinical environment a questionable therapeutic practice.

A less direct but more valid approach to integrating traditional research findings with clinical practice involves relating the results back to a particular theoretical framework and then allowing the theory, which has been supported by research, to guide therapeutic practice. Burr et al. (1973, p. 19) refer to this approach as the "theoretical method" and describe it as "the process of going from technical research literature to 'theory' and from theory to practice rather than trying to directly apply research literature to practical situations." This means that when a therapist encounters a particular practice problem in the clinical environment, the preferred procedure is to translate that problem into a question related to theory and to derive the solution from a theoretical analysis, rather than to seek the solution directly from a specific study based on traditional research procedures. An unsupported or unverified theory is of limited clinical use to the practicing therapist. The role of traditional deductive empirical research is congruent with the "theoretical method" described by Burr et al. (1973). The researcher typically develops a hypothesis or "prediction" based on some theoretical perspective and then submits the hypothesis to an empirical examination. If the investigator's research hypothesis is supported, the researcher has provided another piece of evidence supporting the theory. If the research hypothesis is not supported, the theory may have to be modified or revised. This interaction between traditional experimental research and theory is well established in many fields in the behavioral and biomedical sciences.

The value of research literature in the ''theoretical method'' is obviously related to the evidence it provides for or against a particular theoretical position. Thus, if the results of several research studies support a particular theoretical position, the therapist can feel relatively confident about applying treatment procedures based on the theory to solve a particular practice problem. For example, the practice of splinting to reduce upper extremity hypertonus in individuals who have suffered a cerebrovascular accident is controversial. The controversy is related to several different theoretical perspectives. One school of thought argues for splinting, while another argues against it (Trombly, 1982). Some proponents of splinting advocate the use of static splints over dynamic splints, while others debate the value of dorsal over volar splints in reducing upper extremity spasticity. Each of these viewpoints is based on a theoretical interpretation of how the neuromotor system, including muscle spindles and alpha motor neurons, functions in normal and disordered states. Without the advantage of a body of empirical evidence, it is impossible to ascertain which theoretical interpretation of neuromotor function is correct and, therefore, which therapeutic practice is the most effective. McPherson et al. (1982) recently attempted to provide some research data to help resolve the ''theoretical'' controversy associated with the use of volar versus dorsal resting hand splints as a treatment to reduce hypertonus. They randomly assigned ten patients with upper extremity spasticity to two treatment conditions. Members of one group received a volar resting hand splint, while members of the other group were fitted with a dorsal resting hand splint. The degree of upper extremity hypertonicity was measured with a spring-weighted scale before, during, and after splinting. The final results revealed no statistically significant difference in reduction of spasticity between the two groups. Thus, neither the theoretical position supporting dorsal splinting nor the theoretical position advocating volar splinting was empirically supported. If, on the other hand, the results had confirmed the use of volar splinting over dorsal splinting, the theoretical interpretation of why volar splinting reduces spasticity would have been strengthened. If additional investigators conducted subsequent studies that replicated this finding under several different conditions and with a variety of different samples, the theoretical position would gradually become more established. After enough supportive evidence was provided through numerous research studies, certain guidelines or parameters would be developed and refined and the theoretical position would become a generally accepted guide for practice.

The ''theoretical method'' of integrating traditional research and clinical practice clearly illustrates the crucial nexus between theory testing and development and traditional research. Therapeutic practice based on a synthesis of theory and research provides a firm foundation for clinical intervention that is removed from trial and error or intuition. It should also be obvious from the previous discussion that this is a complex process of interaction which generally continues over a long period of time.

The argument could be made that differential roles for treatment evaluation based on single system designs and traditional group-comparison research are evolving. The small-N procedures serve best to monitor and evaluate practice on an individual, day-to-day basis, while traditional group-comparison procedures are best suited for selection of intervention programs for a particular handicapped population which are based on demonstrated evidence of overall effectiveness.

The relationship between single system designs and traditional group-comparison research methods suggests a potentially useful model for developing knowledge related to clinical practice. Several successful replications of a small-N study focusing on a specific issue or problem may provide the basis for a traditional group-comparison investigation. Single system designs can be used to provide the initial data for generating theoretical hypotheses for large-N experimental research; the successful replication of several small-N evaluation studies would indicate a reasonable basis for expecting a successful outcome from a large-N group-comparison research investigation. The combined results of small-N and group-comparison research can demonstrate the empirical effectiveness of a treatment program and help establish a practice that is scientifically based.

Prior to the elaboration of specific evaluation procedures, it may be instructive to provide a brief, discipline-oriented perspective concerning evaluation activities in clinical environments. The remaining chapters provide therapists with much information on the technical aspects of evaluating and measuring clinical change. This material emphasizes the *how* of evaluation but does not address the equally important issues of *why* we evaluate and *what* should be evaluated. Without consideration of these factors, the how of evaluation is devoid of context and can become a sterile clinical exercise. To understand why we evaluate what we do requires that we explore the rationale or ''philosophy'' behind our more commonly employed intervention procedures and how that philosophy influences the practice of evaluating client performance.

Discipline Perspectives and Professional Belief Systems

There has been much professional discussion and debate regarding the nature of a discipline. It is patently obvious that there are vast differences between many disciplines (medicine, psychology, education, etc.). What is seldom noted is that there are also a number of similarities. For example, many of the problems faced by occupational and physical therapy researchers are similar to those encountered by researchers in medicine, psychology, and sociology. In some cases the specific context or content may differ, but viewed broadly, the problems are quite similar. Within several disciplines, there are ongoing and vigorous debates concerning philosophical approaches to research and measurement and concerning preferred methodologies, and there is the perennial debate regarding applied versus basic research. If various professionals are to profit from the advances of science in general, it is important to explore various disciplinary differences and similarities regarding the general character and nature of research and evaluation, the methodologies used, and the fundamental views regarding research and evaluation held by various professional groups.

It is neither feasible nor productive to discuss discipline perspectives related to numerous fields of study. The purpose of this section is illustrative rather than exhaustive. The differing philosophical orientations of one specific discipline are contrasted with those commonly associated with occupational and physical therapy, and the implications for research and evaluation are briefly discussed.

By review of the techniques, perspectives, and problems associated with various fields, much can be learned regarding the general evaluative process. All too often one's perception of a problem and the approach used to examine that problem are unnecessarily narrowed by a single, insular disciplinary focus or by what may be referred to as a professional belief system.

The professional belief system or ''value system'' of most health related practitioners, including physical and occupational therapists, has been strongly influenced by what is generally referred to as the medical model. The academic and clinical education and training of occupational and physical therapists is strongly influenced by the medical model, and therapists generally practice in clinical environments such as hospitals or rehabilitation centers with strong medical model orientations.

The medical model orientation is one example of a basic professional belief system. The professional belief system as defined here refers to the individual's basic philosophic orientation concerning what should be done in order to effectively treat a person with any type of disabling condition. In a very superficial sense the medical model posits an underlying etiology that acts on or affects various organs, systems, or internal processes and thereby results in certain physical or psychological symptoms. The logic on which the traditional medical model is based is to diagnose or discover the underlying basis of the client's symptoms and then to direct therapy toward the "cause" of the disorder. Direct treatment of symptoms is not the therapeutic method of choice. Prophylactic measures aimed at relieving the symptoms while eschewing the "nature" of the disorder are considered acceptable only when the cause is unknown or believed undiscoverable. Obviously, a professional belief system such as that associated with the medical model will influence the particular treatment strategy used with a given client and will determine what specific behaviors and skills will be evaluated to ascertain whether the intervention was effective.

Different disciplines often exhibit different professional belief systems. In some disciplines, various subgroups within the same discipline may adopt different professional orientations or belief systems. The professional belief systems of various disciplines may be complementary or contradictory. For example, many special educators and psychologists are adamantly opposed to interventions and evaluations based on the logic of the medical model (Kauffman and Hallahan, 1974). Instead, their professional belief systems may be based on an ecological inventory and/or task analysis model. This model emphasizes functional content rather than underlying causes or their related processes. This particular perspective stresses an environmentally relevant description of the client's current functional level and attempts remediation through compensatory strategies based on task analysis and often set in a behavioral paradigm. The "cause" of a particular dysfunction is not of direct remedial concern, nor is diagnostic testing deemed a necessary prerequisite to intervention.

Although the previous description of professional belief systems and dichotomous intervention models is oversimplified and superficial, it highlights the basic philosophical differences that may exist between disciplines. An example may serve to illustrate further the distinction between professional belief systems and how they may influence treatment and evaluation. Assume that the client under discussion is a 7-year-old boy with severe perceptual and coordination problems but no overt physical, motor, or sensory deficits. Let us assume further that the ability to button has been identified by the parent as an important daily living skill for the child to learn. Presently, the child is unable to accomplish any type of buttoning task due to his perceptual and coordination problems. A therapist with a *behavioral* orientation (professional belief system) may begin remediation by breaking the task down into its component parts, identifying the environments in which the skill will be used, and then setting up a contingency management program in which the child is reinforced for completing the successive tasks leading to buttoning. The particular skills that the therapist chooses to teach and evaluate will obviously be closely related to the behaviorally oriented intervention program he or she has developed. On the other hand, a therapist with a professional belief system based on *medical model* logic might begin intervention by administering several diagnostic tests to determine the underlying cause of the child's poor perception and coordination. Following the diagnostic assessment the therapist may conclude that the child has apraxia with accompanying tactile or somatosensory deficits. The therapist has identified an underlying process (praxis) which is deficient. A series of treatment activities are then prescribed to help remediate the underlying dysfunction. When the "cause" of the dysfunction is ameliorated, the child's coordination will be improved and he will be able to perform tasks, such as buttoning, that require a high degree of motor skill. The therapist following a medical model will evaluate a different set of skills or abilities than the therapist advocating a behavioral approach, even though the ultimate goal of both therapists is similar. The therapist who bases intervention on the logic of the medical model may argue that the contingency management procedure based on task analysis is only treatment of a symptom and thus the teaching of a "splinter skill" which will not generalize. The therapist using the behavioral approach might counter that he or she taught the child a functional skill that was identified as important in the child's environment and that this skill was taught in the most effective manner possible.

The implications of various professional belief systems on the choice of treatment and the way that treatment is evaluated should be obvious. Therapists working in various clinical settings, particularly those employed in nontraditional environments such as school systems, need to be aware of the influence professional orientations can have on the planning and interpretation of treatment evaluation. Regardless of the specific professional belief system held by the therapist or of the intervention strategy advocated, however, evaluation of the results of intervention in the most effective and systematic manner possible is necessary. If this is accomplished and the results of the intervention are beneficial to the client, the therapist can be confident that his or her professional belief system is a therapeutically useful one and that interventions based on that belief system are capable of producing the desired effect. It is clear from the previous discussion that differing theoretical orientations or professional belief systems influence practice. They will directly determine the assessment or measurement tool used, the intervention strategy implemented, and the behaviors or skills to be evaluated. At the same time, the evaluation methodologies that are described in later chapters are theory free. They are designed to provide the clinician with a systematic method of evaluating treatment effectiveness regardless of theoretical predisposition, and this is an important point to bear in mind throughout the upcoming chapters.

AN INTRODUCTION TO
_____ TREATMENT EVALUATION _____

If Aristotle's maxim to "define your terms" is to be followed, it is appropriate to begin with a simple definition of treatment evaluation or evaluation research. The two terms are used interchangeably throughout the text. Treatment evaluation is defined here as the *systematic application of applied research procedures in assessing the design, implementation and effectiveness of therapeutic intervention programs*. Treatment evaluation as described and elaborated in the following chapters involves the use of applied and field research methodologies to assess the effectiveness and efficiency of therapeutic strategies employed by occupational and physical therapists.

It should be emphasized that this definition does not imply that evaluation procedures should follow any specified or particular combination of research methods. In fact, in subsequent chapters the argument is made that many of the more traditional research methodologies including pretest-posttest group-comparisons and traditional "experimental" designs are often inappropriate for the evaluation of therapeutic change. Treatment evaluation is considered a "clinical" activity, and as such, its practitioners include clinical therapists as well as academicians and researchers, and its methods may cover the gamut of applied research paradigms. The evaluation approaches that are presented in this text are *systematic* to the extent that they employ basic procedures for gathering valid, reliable evidence designed to determine the extent of clinical change in persons receiving therapy services.

Differences between treatment evaluation, treatment research and more traditional empirical procedures have existed for many years. Early considerations of this topic often seemed to be unproductive and characterized more by rhetoric than by serious examination (Cook and Reichardt, 1979). Some progress has been made in recent years, however, and a brief initial discussion of the issues appears warranted to place both traditional and evaluation research in some degree of perspective.

In many situations the distinctions between evaluation and traditional research are minimal, if they exist at all. In fact, Hemphill (1969, p. 189) posed the question of whether or not evaluation should "be considered simply a subset of the more general set of activities denoted by the term 'research'." For the serious student who wishes to pursue a more detailed study of the topic, it will soon become evident that this question remains relevant to some degree even today.

One of the distinctions between traditional research and evaluation involves the generic purpose for which such an effort is initiated. Cronbach

(1982) observes that evaluation is presumably undertaken to generate information for making decisions. Such decisions might pertain to selecting the most effective treatment procedure or modality. Evaluation may also address whether the treatment technique is effective. These purposes obviously involve questions of immedate utility. For example, does the application of paraffin result in increased range of motion in the affected joints of a 65-year-old patient with rheumatoid arthritis? Does the introduction of a commercially available seat cushion result in a decrease in the incidence of decubiti and related skin irritation in a person with a cervical spinal cord injury? Answers to these and other related clinical concerns are sought to solve immediate problems. The answers to such questions are a fundamental purpose of treatment evaluation efforts. Some traditional research efforts also share this purpose. Most "applied" or "field" research identify similar, if not identical, goals. The broader concept of experimental and quasi-experimental research, however, includes other purposes, such as the development and testing of specific theoretical predictions or hypotheses. The immediate practical application of clinical knowledge is generally a secondary consideration in most traditional research paradigms.

The preceding comments may indicate that evaluation can be considered to be synonymous with applied research approaches. This notion was proposed by Stake and Denny (1969), although they were somewhat tentative in their assertion and suggested that more was actually involved. Stake and Denny (1969, p. 374) described evaluation as a form of applied research and identified the principal difference between traditional research and evaluation as "the degree to which the findings are generalizable beyond their application to a given product, program or locale." Certainly this is a prominent distinction, since traditional empirical research in which group-comparison methods are employed and random selection and assignment of participants are emphasized places a premium on generalizability. Treatment evaluation, as defined here and elaborated in subsequent chapters, focuses on the immediate situation and client needs and places a relatively lower priority on the ability to generalize the particular findings to a "population." The emphasis is placed on developing procedures and methodology designed to demonstrate the effectiveness of therapeutic procedures applied to a given client in a specific therapeutic situation.

Recent advances in evaluation methodology have tended to exacerbate the distinction between traditional research and evaluation (cf. Anderson and Ball, 1978; Cronbach, 1982; Popham, 1974). It appears inevitable that the differences will continue to widen and that the concepts of generalizability and the immediate utility of the results will no longer be viewed as the principal distinguishing factors between traditional research and evaluation methodology. An attempt is made to establish some functional distinctions between "pure" treatment, treatment evaluation, treatment research, and "pure" research in the final chapter of the text. To try and make these distinctions prior to presenting the specific material on treatment evaluation and research strategies would be premature.

Types of Evaluation

In various professional circles there are differences of opinion regarding the precise parameters of evaluation. From one perspective, any information obtained by any means and pertaining to the implementation or outcome of a treatment is considered a type of evaluation. This perspective is so broad that any resulting definition fails to limit the boundaries for evaluation activities. This orientation fosters a "common sense" approach to evaluating program outcomes. Although there certainly is a place for common sense judgments in evaluation, they should not be considered a formal method of treatment evaluation. Common sense evaluations can lead to faulty conclusions, and a more systematic approach is obviously needed.

Another type of judgment often referred to as evaluation is an assessment of whether certain activities are in conformity with generally accepted professional standards. Evaluations of many health care and rehabilitation programs are based, in part, on compliance to certain professional standards commonly accepted in the field. For example, a rehabilitation program may be judged or "evaluated" on the basis of a therapist-to-client ratio. Current standards may be invoked to dictate that an "adequate" program must have a given therapist-to-client ratio.

In many instances, professional standards that are used to evaluate a program are not based on empirical evidence. Rather, they embody a tradition and the dictates of long-standing practice. For example, there is little scientific evidence linking therapist-patient ratios to treatment effectiveness, yet this criterion may be used to assess the worth of a rehabilitation program and may lead to increases or decreases in financial and manpower resources.

Another activity often regarded as evaluative in clinical settings consists of superficial, impressionistic judgments of therapy effectiveness. These judgments are often justified as being based on "clinical expertise" or "clinical experience." An experienced therapist may assess the effectiveness of a new wheelchair design by observing a few settings in which the new chair is used and by judging whether what occurs is better, the same, or worse than what the therapist regards as "usual" wheelchair performance on the basis of past experience. Although assessments based on clinical expertise have attractive features of being inexpensive and easy to perform, they frequently are inadequate as methods of providing data designed to guide programmatic decisions. Clinical impressions in a variety of applied fields are known to vary widely from judge to judge (Rossi and Freeman, 1982). In addition, such judgments are often made without respect to critical considerations regarding the individual characteristics of clients or the uniqueness of various situations. In short, unsystematic clinical judgments often can be erroneous or misleading.

Increasingly, administrators and program directors responsible for making program decisions are demanding more than ''common sense'' assessments of program effectiveness or evaluations based on clinical expertise. They are requiring more objective and systematic measures of program outcome in order to justify ever-increasing financial and manpower commitments.

Rossi and Freeman (1982) identify four types of systematic evaluation activity. The first type of evaluation relates to gathering and developing information for *program planning*. The second form of evaluation concerns strategies for *monitoring program implementation*, while the third type of evaluation deals with assessing *program impact*. The fourth and final form of evaluation described by Rossi and Freeman (1982) is designed to determine *program efficiency*. This last type of evaluation deals with determining cost-benefit ratios and evaluating how efficiently program resources were employed.

A comprehensive evaluation of a new program should include all four types of evaluation activity. Rossi and Freeman (1982) note, however, that for some programs, particularly those already established and operating, not all four types of evaluation are possible or necessary. The focus of this text is on the third type of evaluation activity—assessing *program impact*. The reader is referred to the works of Cronbach (1982), Rossi and Freeman (1982), and others for more detailed information on conducting evaluations related to program planning, program implementation and program efficiency.

Program Impact Evaluation

As stated previously, the focus of this text is on procedures and methods of assessing treatment impact, particularly program impact on individual clients. An impact evaluation is designed to gauge the extent to which a treatment produces changes in the desired direction. It implies that there is a set of predetermined, specifically defined therapeutic objectives. A treatment that has impact is one that achieves some movement or change toward the desired objectives. These objectives may be behavioral or social, such as developing the ability to live in a group home environment, or they may be biological or physical, such as a reduction in spasticity or an increase in upper extremity strength.

A plan for collecting, organizing and analyzing information is required to conduct an impact evaluation. The plan or design allows the evaluator to demonstrate in a persuasive systematic manner that any changes which occurred were a function of the particular treatment and cannot be easily explained in other ways. Specific impact assessment design may vary considerably, depending on the nature of the intervention and the setting in which it occurs. Sometimes it is possible to use traditional experimental designs in which there are control and treatment groups that receive different therapeutic programs and are constructed through randomization (Cook and Campbell, 1979). In much clinical evaluation, however, it is often more productive to employ nontraditional procedures rather than classic true or quasi experiments. As is demonstrated in Chapters 2 and 3, it is usually difficult or impossible to employ randomized experiments in most clinical settings. As a result, nontraditional research designs, particularly those involving a small number of individuals referred to throughout the text as small-N or single system designs, will be advocated as an individualized method for evaluating treatment impact. In later chapters the argument is made that with proper safeguards and appropriate qualifications, single system designs can provide firm and convincing evidence regarding treatment effects. In addition, such designs are often more appropriate for use in clinical settings than are the more widely used group-comparison research procedures.

CONCLUSION

The major premise of this book is that systematically planned and conducted evaluation will result in a clinical practice that is therapeutically effective and valued by the consumers of occupational and physical therapy services. Conducting well-conceived and properly executed treatment evaluation and then building the results of those evaluations into future treatments and programming will greatly enhance clinical practice. The arena of clinical practice is of primary concern to us as therapists, for it is here that we have an impact on the lives of others. The process of treatment evaluation should be viewed as a vital adjunct to validate and guide clinical practice, not as an end in itself. Treatment evaluation, if properly applied, can be adapted to meet the needs of multiple practice settings while standards of precision, accuracy and objectivity are maintained. These standards will help ensure the professional and empirical integrity of the disciplines in which they are employed.

The small-N single system designs and related procedures that are presented in the remaining chapters can be integrated with almost any framework for practice or with any theoretical orientation. The clinician does not have to subscribe to any particular conception of practice in order to profit from the systematic evaluation methods that single system designs offer. The use of these procedures will eventually facilitate the synthesis of research, evaluation and clinical practice. As a result, therapists will become more objective and scientific in their approach to intervention.

Therapists employing evaluation strategies will conduct their practice as a problem-solving exercise, an exercise in which they assume little and view their function as that of a clinical investigator whose goal is to find out if a treatment is effective for a given client. In order to accomplish this task, the therapist will systematically monitor and evaluate practice outcomes with each client, using the appropriate procedure. The intervention methods employed will be grounded, to the maximum extent possible, in empirically based knowledge validated by both traditional research procedures and evaluation methods. Those intervention strategies not displaying such support should be used with appropriate caution.

CHAPTER 2

Traditional Research Methods: The Group-Comparison Approach

INTRODUCTION

Occupational and physical therapists must base their clinical practice on a body of reliable theory and facts if they wish to be considered true rehabilitation professionals. Reliable theory and facts are not easily obtained; they are established through the time-consuming processes of scientific investigation. A common approach to verifying theory and establishing reliable factual data is the experimental method. Although this method is familiar to most readers, it is reviewed here in its simplest form.

The experimental method associated with large-N research has been the standard against which all other methods have been compared for the last several decades. Basically, the group-comparison experimental method consists of a contrast between two conditions. The individuals in both of these conditions are treated identically, except for one feature that is different. This difference is referred to as the treatment or, more commonly, the independent variable. The designation of ''independent'' stresses that the manipulation of the variable (treatment) is under the control of the investigator. Some aspect of performance for the participants in the two conditions is measured and recorded after the treatment has been administered. The critical feature of participant performance is referred to as the dependent variable, criterion variable, or outcome variable. Any difference between the two conditions that the investigator observes on the dependent variable is called the treatment effect and is usually assumed to have been produced or "caused" by the experimental intervention. A hypothesis of causal relationship in traditional experimental research asserts that a particular characteristic or occurrence is one of the factors that determines another characteristic or occurrence. In classic deductive hypothesis testing, the hypothesis represents a theoretical prediction based on some conceptual model or theoretical perspective. For example, a researcher may develop a hypothesis concerning the efficacy of heat as treatment for increasing range of motion (ROM) in the extremities of patients with arthritis. This hypothesis is derived from a larger theoretical framework concerning how heat affects muscle, connective tissue, and related joint structures. The investigator may hypothesize that treatment with heat, administered via a paraffin bath, will increase the upper extremity ROM in patients with restricted joint range due to rheumatoid arthritis (RA). In a traditional experimental test of this hypothesis the researcher would arrange for a number of subjects diagnosed as having RA and reduced upper extremity ROM to receive a daily treatment with paraffin and for a number of comparable subjects *not* to receive any form of heat therapy during the period of the experiment. In other words, the investigator would "select" the subjects to be assigned to different conditions or treatments. In one condition, the subjects would be exposed to the treatment (the paraffin bath), and in the alternate condition, the subjects would receive a different form of standard therapy that did not involve heat. Technically, this would be referred to as manipulating the independent variable. The investigator would assign the subjects to the different conditions in such a way as to ensure that the two groups did not differ, except by chance, before they received the respective interventions. Comparison of the upper extremity ROM of the participants in the two conditions, after one group had received the paraffin treatment and the other had not, would provide evidence demonstrating whether applying heat led to an increase in upper extremity mobility. An empirical relationship between the independent and the dependent variable may be established by keeping careful records of the amount of time exposed to treatment and the temperature of the paraffin bath and by carefully recording the joint ROM. Equating these two groups before they have received any intervention lends assurance that they did not differ in some manner that might have led to a subsequent difference in joint ROM. In addition, the experimenter might introduce "controls" to protect against the possibility that different experiences during the intervention, other than the paraffin baths, might be responsible for a difference in joint ROM. For example, the researcher might see to it that the amount of pain-reducing medication taken by all the subjects did not increase or decrease during the period of the study.

The researcher is not primarily interested in describing the performance of the *individual* participants in the specific treatment and control conditions. Rather, the main objective is to make some inferences about the behavior or performance of other similar individuals suffering from RA who have not participated in the study. For instance, in the example previously described, the researcher would like to generalize his findings from the individuals with arthritis who took part in the study to other similar individuals who also are affected by RA. Rarely will the researcher be able to test or treat all the possible "subjects." Obviously, the investigator would not be able to include all the individuals with RA in a particular city or state into his or her study. Instead, the researcher selects a sample of individuals from a larger group or population and administers the treatment to some individuals in the sample and then makes inferences about the effect the treatment would have on members of the population based on the experimental outcome.

We refer to the larger group as the population. Members of any population are identified by a set of rules of membership. A sample consists of a smaller set of "elements" drawn from the population. In order to generalize results back to the population, the researcher must randomly select participants comprising the sample from the population (see Figure 2.1.)

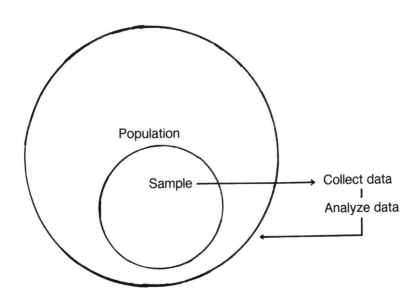

Figure 2.1. Relationship of population, sample, and statistics. A sample is selected from some target population, and data are collected and analyzed. Inferential statistics are used to determine the probability that results based on data from the sample are the same results which would have been obtained if information was collected from the entire population.

When a traditional group-comparison experiment such as the one described previously is possible, it has been considered the most powerful and effective method of testing the hypothesis that one variable causally influences another variable. The basic outline of such an experiment is relatively simple. An "experimental" or treatment group is exposed to an assumed causal (independent) variable, while a "control" group is not; the two groups are then compared in terms of the assumed effect (dependent variable). This procedure or methodology allows for the collection of three major types of evidence relevant to testing hypotheses about causal relationships: (1) evidence of concomitant variation, i.e., that the causal (independent) variable and the dependent variable are associated; (2) evidence that the dependent variable did not occur before the causal variable; and (3) evidence ruling out other factors as possible determining conditions of the dependent variable (Cook and Campbell, 1979).

In the traditional group-comparison experiment, evidence of the first type—concomitant variation—is provided very easily. The investigator knows which subjects have been exposed to the treatment or intervention. The researcher simply measures all of the subjects in a systematic way in terms of their performance on the dependent variable (upper extremity range of motion in the previous example) and then determines whether an increase in the dependent measure occurs more often in the subjects who have been exposed to the experimental intervention (paraffin baths in the previous example) than among those who have not received the intervention. This determination is usually made with the assistance of statistical procedures that allow the investigator to compare the average performance of individuals in the two conditions.

Evidence of the second type—that the assumed effect did not occur before the assumed cause—is secured in a couple of different ways. First, the experimental and control groups are set up in such a way that it is reasonable to assume that they did not differ in terms of the dependent variable before exposure to the independent (treatment) variable. Second, the performance of these groups on the dependent variable is measured before exposure to the independent variable. In our hypothetical example, the investigator might randomly assign the participants to the treatment condition (paraffin bath) and the control condition (non-paraffin bath) so that it is reasonable to assume that the subjects in the two groups were comparable in upper extremity joint range of motion before they had received any intervention. An alternative procedure would be to administer a pretest of joint range of motion at the beginning of the study to determine the upper extremity joint range of motion and then to equate the two groups based on their scores on this pretest. Since the hypothesis asserts that the use of heat (the paraffin bath) will lead to the acquisition of an increase in joint range of motion, what needs to be demonstrated is that the experimental group should not have more joint range than the control group before the start of the intervention. This requirement does not mean that the subjects who participate in the study must have not had any previous treatment designed to improve upper extremity mobility. It means simply that the two groups should be relatively equal in upper extremity joint range of motion prior to any intervention.

Evidence of the third type—that other factors are ruled out as possible determining conditions or agents—is a very important one in the traditional control-group research paradigm. Ruling out such factors ensures the *internal validity* of the experiment.

Campbell and Stanley (1963) argue that internal validity is the absolute minimum without which any experimental manipulation becomes uninterpretable. They (1963, p. 5) contend that an investigation can be said to be internally valid when convincing evidence is provided to answer the following question: "Did in fact the experimental treatments make a difference in this specific experimental instance?" Within the ·clinical research model the question is whether or not the change in client performance was caused by the treatment. To the extent that alternative explanations can be offered as evidence contributing to or causing clinical change, the internal validity of the study under consideration is weakened.

THREATS TO INTERNAL VALIDITY

Campbell and Stanley (1963) originally identified several major sources of secondary variation that can produce internal invalidity in an investigation. These sources of invalidity represent alternative factors or variables other than the treatment (independent variable) that may have produced a difference between the two groups on the outcome measure. Obviously, it is to the investigator's advantage to rule out or control for as many of these sources of invalidity as possible. The degree of confidence that the investigator can have regarding whether the treatment was the "cause" of any observed effects is directly related to the extent to which the various sources of internal invalidity can be controlled. The traditional "true" experiment described by Campbell and Stanley (1963) is generally considered the most effective method of controlling various threats to internal validity. Additional sources of internal invalidity have been identified since Campbell and Stanley's (1963) seminal work in this area (Cook and Campbell, 1979). The original threats identified by Campbell and Stanley (1963), however, are widely recognized as the most serious sources of invalidity in traditional empirical investigations. These threats include history, maturation, testing, statistical regression, experimental motality, interaction effects, instrumentation, selection, and experimenter bias.

History

History refers to any single event or series of events which occur between a set of observations or measurements, in addition to the treatment being evaluated. For example, if during the interval between pretest and posttest the intervention site was changed, a new therapist took over the treatment program, or a concurrent intervention was introduced (e.g., the use of a new drug), these events become plausible explanations for any changes observed in the client's behavior if they were not controlled for or ruled out by the design.

Maturation

Maturation may be defined as biological, physiological, or psychological changes that occur over a period of time and are due primarily to growth or adaptation. Imagine that a treatment program consisting of some form of progressive resistive exercise is given to a group of five adolescents with Down's syndrome to improve their physical strength. The students are tested at the beginning of the program and again 10 months later. At the second testing it is found that the youngsters are stronger than they were when initially tested 10 months earlier. From this particular example, in which only one group was evaluated with a pretest and a posttest, it is readily apparent that changes caused by experience and maturation were not adequately controlled. Would the increase in strength observed at the posttest have occurred if the students had not been enrolled in the treatment program? Maturation may be as valid a reason for the increase in strength as the treatment. Maturation effects are generally controlled for by designs that include both a treatment and control or comparison group. Effects due to maturation will show up in both conditions, and any difference between the groups can then be more accurately related to the intervention received by the treatment group.

Testing

In an attempt to carry out a before-and-after comparison, investigators often administer pretests to subjects before the independent variable or intervention is administered. Sometimes, because of the pretest, subjects score differently on the posttest than they would have if no pretest had been given. When an individual is administered an assessment of motor skills for the second time (posttest), there is a high probability that the second score will be different from the initial score. In such a case, testing may be a source of internal invalidity and influence performance on the dependent measure. When the same or similar test is administered a second time without controls, the higher scores might be attributable, at least in part, to the repeated testing.

Pretests may also "sensitize" the respondents to the particular variable or intervention under investigation. Suppose an investigator was studying the attitudes of therapists toward state licensure. Prior to interviewing the therapists on their individual views, the investigator has the respondents fill out a questionnaire about licensure and certification issues. This pretest questionnaire may influence or bias the respondents' views on licensure, so that any attitudes expressed after filling out the questionnaire may not be representative. Invalidity produced by such testing effects is generally controlled for by use of an experimental design that includes at least one nonpretested control group.

Statistical Regression

Another threat to internal validity related to testing is statistical regression. A fundamental principle of statistical inference is that in repeated testing both extremely high and extremely low scores within an overall range of possible scores will tend to be pulled toward the mean as testing is repeated. If the first time that a person takes a particular test his or her score is at the *extreme end* of the scale of possible scores, i.e., either a very high score or a very low score, the second time that person takes the same test the score is likely to move toward the mean or average. In other words, an individual scoring high or low on a test tends to score closer to the mean on a successive test. This tendency for scores to migrate toward the mean is termed statistical regression (see Figure 2.2).

Physical and occupational therapy investigators often deal with clients whose performance is very low. Indeed, subjects are frequently selected because of their extremely poor performance on a particular test. For example, a group of infants with Down's syndrome may be selected for a program of early intervention based on their low scores on the *Bayley Scales of Infant Development* (Bayley, 1969). A program of intervention may be initiated, and following a period of treatment, the infants would be retested. The extremely low scores of some of the infants would improve (move closer to the mean) as a result of statistical regression, not as a result of any specific intervention. To control for this statistical artifact, the investigator could divide those infants with poor scores into treatment and comparison groups and observe the resulting differences between them.

Experimental Mortality

Loss of subjects or clients by attrition or simple discontinued performance during experimentation obviously can affect comparisons between groups. Such a loss may invalidate the entire study, particularly if

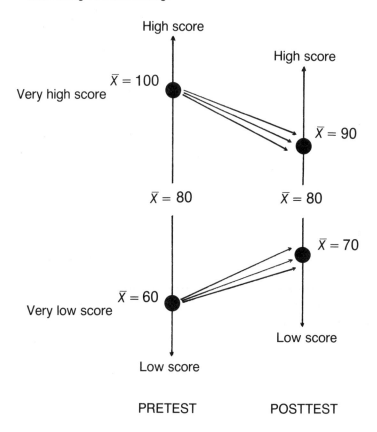

Figure 2.2. Schematic diagram of statistical regression phenomenon. (Adapted from: Huck, S. W., Cormier, W. H., and Bounds, W. G. (1974). *Reading statistics and research.* New York, Harper & Row, p. 237.)

some component of the treatment or intervention results in a systematic loss of individuals from the treatment condition. If analysis of results is still possible, it will be more difficult with uneven groups due to attrition, and specific statistical adjustments will have to be made to compensate for samples that become uneven due to subject attrition.

Instrumentation

A seventh threat to internal validity is instrumentation. Instrumentation refers to the effect any change in the observational technique or measurement instrument might have on the dependent measure. Obviously, any mechanical device may need servicing, may malfunction, or may become unreliable. The problem of instrumentation also becomes crucial when human beings are used as judges, observers, raters, coders, interviewers or graders of client behavior or performance. The difference between a treatment and a control group may have occurred because observers or raters (1) become more experienced over time, (2) become fatigued, (3) learn about the purpose of the study, or (4) become more relaxed or more stringent in evaluating performance. Differences between the two conditions may also occur if the investigator uses different observers or raters for pretesting and posttesting.

Selection

Another source of invalidity for a group-comparison study is selection. The investigator cannot be certain that the two groups are equivalent unless the clients are randomly assigned to the treatment and control groups, which thus gives each client an equal chance of being selected in either group. Selection becomes a problem whenever clients who voluntarily seek exposure to the treatment are compared with clients who do not seek exposure. Significant differences resulting from such a study could then be the consequence of nonequivalent groups rather than of the treatment or independent variable.

Selection may also involve the threat of statistical regression if extreme scores are used to select clients for inclusion in a treatment group but not in the control group (as might be the case in studies concerning the effect of remediation on handicapped populations).

Experimenter Bias

Recently, concern has grown over the total effect of experimenter bias on an experimental situation. Rosenthal (1966) pioneered in demonstrating that an investigator's expectations regarding subject performance may influence the data gathered. His work revealed that preconceived expectations regarding the performance of specific students influenced how teachers rated the students in classroom situations. Subsequent studies revealed that teacher expectation of student performance constrained or dictated the teacher's actions toward a student in subtle ways. These actions, in turn, elicited the "expected" reaction from the student. Although this phenomenon has not been formally demonstrated in clinical settings, it is reasonable to assume that experimenter expectancies exist in any setting. It is well known that the expectation of an investigator, though it may be unconscious and unintended, may affect the data gathered. A blind recording procedure is often employed to control for the effect of experimenter bias. In a blind procedure, the investigator who is responsible for recording subject performance is unaware of or "blind" to which clients are in the treatment group and which clients are in the control condition. Thus, the investigator's expectation that subjects in the treatment group will outperform subjects in the control group will not affect the recording of the dependent measure.

CONTROLLING THREATS TO INTERNAL VALIDITY

Maintaining or establishing the internal validity of an investigation has been viewed as absolutely essential in the conduct of traditional large-N group-comparison research. Much energy has been expended in the development of sophisticated design procedures and statistical techniques to help ensure the internal validity of a study. Robinson (1976) has identified five basic procedures designed to control for the effect or influence of secondary variables and thereby ensure the internal validity of experimental manipulations:

1. Identify any variables which may act as secondary variables and remove them from the experimental situation altogether.
2. Identify the possible effect of a secondary variable and then use a design that will hold the variable constant for all groups. For example, if an investigator has reason to believe that gender may affect performance on the dependent measure, he or she may decide to hold this variable constant by using only males in the study.
3. Identify possible confounding variables and develop a design in which the secondary variable is considered as another independent or treatment factor.
4. Use random assignment of subjects and procedures to equalize all secondary variables across groups.
5. Finally, the effect of secondary variables may be controlled or partialled out by the use of specific statistical procedures.

Each procedure has its advantages and disadvantages, and although one control procedure may be superior to another in one situation, it may not be superior to another in a different situation. In spite of this qualification, however, one control procedure is routinely advocated as the preferred method and is associated with the most powerful types of group-comparison designs. That procedure is randomization.

Randomization is a procedure for equating groups with respect to secondary or confounding variables. The power of randomization in equating groups was recognized by Fisher (1925) and incorporated as a central aspect of early experimental designs. Randomization does not guarantee that all groups are equal, but groups in which the clients are randomly assigned to treatment or control conditions have a greater probability of being equated than do groups in which subjects or clients are not randomly assigned

(Williams, 1982). Another theoretical principle of randomization is that the larger the number of subjects randomly assigned to groups, the higher the probability that these groups will be relatively equal on all characteristics or parameters. If 500 people are randomly assigned to 10 groups, there is much greater probability that the 10 groups will be equal in terms of various background characteristics than if only 50 people are randomly divided into 10 groups.

Four of the five methods of controlling secondary or confounding variables that may threaten internal validity are only effective if the secondary variable can be identified beforehand. Eliminating a variable, holding it constant, making it an alternative independent variable, or controlling it via statistical adjustment is only possible if the variable that may be a threat can be identified. The major advantage of random assignment is that it equates groups across all possible parameters. Randomization is considered to be the overall best tool for controlling many sources of secondary variation at one time in large-N group-comparison designs. Random assignment can equate groups for all secondary variables, including those not apparent. The reader is referred to one of the many excellent texts on experimental methodology for a more detailed discussion of randomization and other methods used to ensure internal validity (Christensen, 1980; Keppel, 1973; Kerlinger, 1973).

EXTERNAL VALIDITY

The "true" experimental designs and variations to be discussed in the next section have built-in controls for most threats to internal validity. These designs, however, do not have built-in controls for all the various threats to external validity. External validity refers to the extent to which the results of an experiment can be generalized to other subjects or populations and to different environments. In other words, with what clients and under what environmental conditions can the same results be expected? External validity can be classified into two broad types: population validity and ecological validity (Bracht and Glass, 1968). Population validity concerns the generalization of the results to other subjects, while ecological validity concerns the generalization of the results to other settings or environmental conditions.

Some sources of external invalidity are not a function of experimental design and cannot be controlled for by design variations; rather, they may be consequences of an inadequate description of the independent variable or dependent measure or may be due to a poor explanation of procedures and methods of the study. Thus, although most sources of internal invalidity can be controlled by the use of various design features, many sources of external invalidity cannot be controlled by design alone.

Random selection of subjects is the single most effective method of ensuring the generalizability of a study's results. There are two kinds of randomization. One is random assignment of clients to treatment and control conditions. As discussed previously, this type of randomization is an important feature in controlling several of the threats to internal validity. The second type of randomization is random selection of clients from a target population. Random selection is concerned with selection of subjects or clients who are representative of a population of interest. To the degree that an investigator is able to randomly select clients from a target population, he or she is able to ensure the population validity of the study findings. The experimentally accessible population, i.e., the population from which the investigator can select his clients, however, may or may not be the same as the target population to which he or she wishes to have the results generalize. Clinical researchers often emphasize only random assignment, giving almost exclusive consideration to the demands of internal validity and very little consideration to external validity and the ability to generalize the finds to other patients. We have more to say about this subject in a later section.

—— TRADITIONAL EXPERIMENTAL DESIGNS ——

The distinguishing feature of "experimental" designs, as defined by Campbell and Stanley (1963) and elaborated extensively in the behavioral science research literature, is that these designs enable the investigator to rule out most of the threats to internal validity mentioned earlier. A "true" experimental design in which subjects are randomly assigned to treatment and control conditions and the dependent measure is blindly recorded is widely accepted as the most powerful strategy available to empirically separate the influence of the independent variable (treatment) from the various extraneous factors (secondary variables) whose effects might obscure the findings. The "true" experiment allows the investigator to manipulate the independent variable so that a "cause and effect" relationship can be demonstrated. Any extraneous influences that might alter performance on the dependent measure can be controlled, and the control can be accomplished in different ways, depending upon the source of the confound.

As noted previously, the assignment of subjects to conditions on a random basis is the major factor that gives an experiment its "strength." Random assignment significantly reduces the likelihood that any extraneous difference between subjects or clients could account for differential performance on the dependent measure. A schematic example of an experimental design (the pretest/posttest control group design) would be

$R\,O_1\,X\,O_2$ (treatment group)
$R\,O_1\quad O_2$ (control group),

where R indicates that subjects were randomly assigned to the two conditions and O_1 represents an initial observation or measurement (pretest), X represents the intervention or treatment, and O_2 represents the second observation or measurement (posttest). This diagram represents a basic "true" experiment. Many variations of experimental designs are possible (Campbell and Stanley, 1963; Isaac and Michael, 1975; Kirk, 1973). The designs may differ in many specifics but share the general characteristic of a relatively large number of subjects employed in two or more groups or conditions with emphasis on the elimination of most, if not all, threats to internal validity.

Quasi-experimental Designs

Campbell and Stanley (1963) used the term quasi experiments to refer to investigations in which the experimenter could not control important features that would rule out the various threats to internal validity. An investigation is termed quasi-experimental if there is some limitation to full control over extraneous factors or secondary variables.

The most common restriction that makes an investigation a quasi experiment rather than a "true" experiment is the inability to control the assignment of subjects to groups or conditions. Typically, such intact groups as clients in a particular inpatient or outpatient clinic or patients on a specific ward or in a given hospital are used as experimental participants. It is possible, and often likely, that these intact groups differ from each other on various parameters or dimensions relevant to the study prior to implementation of the treatment or independent variable.

Schematically, a typical quasi-experimental design (the pretest/posttest nonequivalent control group design) would be

$O_1\,X\,O_2$ (treatment group)
$O_1\quad O_2$ (control group),

where the values are the same as those presented previously for the true experiment, except for the dashed line which separates the two groups and which indicates that random assignment was not employed and that the groups are considered nonequivalent.

Various authorities argue that quasi experiments still allow the investigator to make inferences about the effects of experimental manipulations. Indeed, as in true experiments, quasi experiments often permit investigators to manipulate variables to assess the effects. In other situations, quasi experiments are studies of naturally occurring variations that are going to happen anyway.

Correlational Designs

Correlational designs refer to investigations of the association between variables that are not manipulated by the researcher. In the typical correlational study, the clients are selected because of some characteristic they possess prior to coming to the study. The purpose of the correlational approach is to estimate the extent to which variables covary or relate to each other.

In a correlational study the different levels of a variable are not obtained through manipulation of a specific variable but rather through selection of individuals with a predetermined characteristic or standing on some measure or trait. Studies completed with the aim of assessing the relationship between such variables as strength, age, IQ, or medical diagnosis and some other measure are correlational. The information obtained in correlational designs has no direct bearing on causal relationships in the same sense that experiments or even some quasi experiments do.

For example, a researcher may believe that prematurity is a factor associated with later learning disabilities in some children. This relationship may be assessed by determining whether a child meets the criterion of prematurity (i.e., gestational age of 37 weeks or less) and then looking at the incidence of later learning disorders. The finding of a positive correlation does not necessarily confirm a causal relationship between prematurity and learning disability. It is possible that some third variable, such as an abnormality in the uterine environment or the diet of the mother, "caused" both the prematurity and the learning problems. It is possible that a number of extraneous third factors could be related to both the prematurity and a child's learning dysfunction.

One variation of a correlational design encountered commonly in clinical settings is the *ex post facto design*. This design is an attempt to improve on a simple correlational approach by ruling out selected variables that may serve as a rival interpretation of the results. This is accomplished by the selection of clients who differ on the variable of interest but who are matched on other variables. The matching procedure is intended to control for or rule out the influence of these other variables. For instance, in the previous example (correlating prematurity with later learning disabilities), selection of subjects on the basis of whether or not they were premature leaves many other variables uncontrolled. Perhaps clients separated on the variable of prematurity versus no prematurity (full-term delivery) differ in another important way, such as social class. This latter variable (social class) may be responsible for later learning impairment. In an attempt to rule out such a variable, an *ex post facto* design might include clients who differ in whether or not they were born prematurely but who are all members of the same social class. In that way, if there is a relationship between prematurity and later diagnosis of learning disability, one can assume that the variable of social class was not the cause of the result, since this variable was held constant across the two groups of premature and full-term births.

The *ex post facto* design is an attempt to narrow the reasons for the interrelationship between two variables that are to be correlated in a study. The correlational nature of the design, however, makes it ultimately inadequate to establish an unequivocal cause-and-effect relationship. Matching clients on secondary variables in an *ex post facto* fashion is not adequate for ruling out other plausible rival interpretations of the results. An investigator can never be sure that a variable omitted from the matching procedure is not the crucial one and might be sufficiently powerful to account for the relationship.

Correlational designs, in general, are inherently subject to threats to internal validity and to rival interpretations of the results. Complete lack of control over subject assignment to conditions means that many factors other than the one assessed could account for any relationships found. Thus, correlational designs are considered weak as a methodology for demonstrating causal relationships and have a limited usefulness as a methodology for documenting clinical change.

ROLE OF STATISTICAL INFERENCE IN GROUP-COMPARISON DESIGNS

The chain of events which underlies statistical hypothesis testing in traditional group-comparison research is summarized in Figure 2.3. This process begins with the formulation of a *research* hypothesis which, in turn, initiates the traditional group-comparison experiment. Suppose that a theory (e.g., the kinesthetic need theory) predicted that a program of tactile stimulation applied to premature infants would facilitate their growth and development. A group-comparison study could be designed to test this prediction. The research hypothesis concerns the testing of a prediction or an expectation based on a developmental theory. Independent samples of subjects would be drawn from a population (preterm infants). The different samples would then be subjected to different treatment conditions, with one group receiving a program of controlled tactile stimulation and the other group receiving standard nursery care for preterm neonates. Finally, some measure of growth or development would be collected. In this case, the weights of the two groups of infants might be recorded by an observer who is unaware of the group placement of the infants.

During the planning of the investigation, the research hypothesis is translated into a statistical or null hypothesis which is evaluated based on the data obtained from the sample. This evaluation or statistical test consists of the administration of a set of decision rules which are also formed before the start of the investigation. Included in the statistical evaluation of the null hypothesis is an indication of the accuracy associated with a decision reached by an application of the rules. The results of the statistical test are then incorporated into the theory that originally initiated the study (see Figure 2.3).

The general role of statistics in group-comparison research is to describe the characteristics of the sample and, more importantly, to assist the researcher in making inferences from the behavior or performance of the sample to the larger target population. The general characteristics of statistical evaluation should be familiar to the reader and are not elaborated on here in much detail. Essentially, in most group-comparison research, statistical evaluation is designed to determine whether a treatment group can be distinguished statistically from a comparison or control group, based on their performance on a dependent measure. Statistical evaluation consists of applying a specific test to determine whether the difference obtained on the dependent measure is likely to have occurred by "chance." Typically a level of confidence or probability is selected as the criterion for determining whether the results are statistically significant. The difference between groups on the dependent measure is assessed with a statistical test that yields a probability value. A statistically significant difference indicates that the probability level is equal to or smaller than the level of

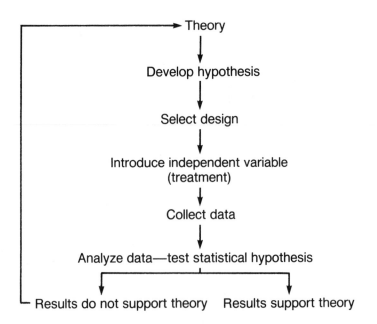

Figure 2.3. Steps in hypothesis testing.

significance or confidence selected. Traditionally, this level of significance has been .05 (Bakan, 1966). If the probability obtained in the study is less than .05, most behavioral science researchers would concede that the difference in performance between the treatment and control group was probably *not* the result of chance but reflected a "true" relationship between the independent and dependent variables (Rosenthal and Rosnow, 1984).

To contend that a relationship is statistically significant does not mean that there is actually a genuine relationship between the variables studied. Even a statistically significant difference could be the result of chance. Chance is the one rival hypothesis that can never be ruled completely out. That is, there may be no relationship between the variables in reality, but there may be a statistically significant difference in the experiment due to the selection of an unusual sample or other factors beyond the researcher's control. This occurrence is referred to as Type I experimental error. The probability of the researcher committing a Type I error is the same as the significance level set by the researcher to reject the null hypothesis. If the significance level is set at .05, there is a 5% chance that the researcher will make a Type I error and reject the null hypothesis when it should have been supported.

The goal of statistical significance testing is to provide a relatively bias-free and consistent method for determining whether a treatment effect is genuine. Indeed, statistical significance is often regarded as the definitive test of whether the independent variable under investigation is important or worth pursuing. Yet statistical significance is not a panacea; it is a function of many different features of an investigation, only one of which is whether there is a "true" relationship between the independent and the dependent variable. Statistical significance is influenced by the size of the sample employed, by the heterogeneity of the subjects, and by the procedures and methods used in a particular investigation. We have more to say about these factors in the next section.

LIMITATIONS OF TRADITIONAL GROUP-COMPARISON DESIGNS

Perhaps the greatest limitation of traditional group-comparison designs as applied to clinical settings is the relatively small number of sufficiently homogeneous clients in most clinical settings that can be included in a research study. Even in large hospitals or institutional settings, variability in age, sex, severity of disorder, etc., limits the selection of clients for any group-comparison study. Other factors, such as medical counterindications and management problems, also play a role in reducing the size of the population from which clients may be selected.

Suppose that an investigator has been fortunate enough to find 20 clients fulfilling the requirements for a comparative evaluation of two treatments of low back pain. The first treatment consists of postural exercises and relaxation techniques. This treatment is considered, based on established use, the standard intervention for low back pain. The second treatment is spinal mobilization. This intervention is considered to have potential, based on preliminary evidence, to reduce the incidence of low back pain. Next, assume that the 20 clients have been selected and randomly assigned into two groups of 10 each; the first group is to receive the standard treatment, and the second group is to receive joint mobilization. For illustrative purposes we will ignore questions of blind recording and reliability of the dependent measure and assume that a valid design has been created. Let us further assume that all 20 of the clients have similar symptoms just prior to intervention and that none of the clients have received either of the treatment programs previously. What we have set up so far is an almost ideal situation from a design standpoint, with one important exception—the *small number* of clients in the study. As noted previously, however, this factor is a typical limitation of clinical research; therefore, it is worth examining some of the statistical inferential processes that are specifically pertinent to this limitation. To this end, let us assume the following outcome for the hypothetical study. Four of 10 clients receiving the standard therapy for low back pain show improvement on some outcome measure related to a reduction in back pain or spinal flexibility, while 8 of 10 clients receiving mobilization evidence a similar degree of improvement. This ratio of 2 to 1 in favor of the mobilization treatment may cause some degree of therapeutic excitement. The investigator may anxiously consult the appropriate set of statistical tables to determine whether the null hypothesis of no difference in effect between the two treatments can be rejected. The researcher may anticipate that the tabled value will contradict the null hypothesis and thereby support mobilization as a better or more effective intervention for low back pain. Alas, the table shows a significance level of about .17, which seems light years away from the much coveted .05 level of significance.

More serious, however, than the investigator's personal disappointment at not establishing a statistically significant result is the error in reasoning which often accompanies the result obtained via statistical hypothesis testing. As noted previously, the essential usefulness of testing for statistical significance is that it provides a relatively objective procedure for determining whether a particular result, such as the difference between two group means, could have been due to chance alone. The failure to obtain a statistically significant result in a group-comparison study, however, does not establish that the observed difference was, in fact, due to chance. Yet statements and attitudes in published reports seem either explicitly or implicitly to convey such an erroneous impression (Bakan, 1966; Carver, 1978). Despite the nonsignificant statistical outcome in the hypothetical example described previously, the 2 to 1 ratio of treatment success for mobilization therapy may have considerable clinical significance if it could be shown to be representative. That is, if it could be replicated and maintained. We are considering, however, the typical clinical situation in which it is generally not possible to increase the sample size in conformity with the maintenance of a given design protocol to determine whether the ratio has both statistical and clinical significance.

Errors that are made in this regard relate to the ''power'' or sensitivity of the statistical manipulations and to the presence of Type II experimental errors in research literatures characterized by small sample sizes and relatively small or medium-sized treatment effects. The concepts of effect size, statistical power and Type II experimental error have been dealt with extensively in previous papers and are beyond the scope of the present discussion (Ottenbacher, 1982, 1984a, 1984b). The point emphasized here is that most group-comparison studies reported in the occupational and the physical therapy research literature are characterized by low power and a high probability of acceptance of a null hypothesis when it should have been rejected (Type II experimental error). One cannot help but wonder how many valuable therapeutic leads may have been lost or ignored when what seemed like a useful clinical treatment effect may have been erroneously interpreted as due to chance (see Ottenbacher et al. (1981) for an example of a study with statistically nonsignificant results that, it was felt, had clinical implications).

Even in those group-comparison designs in which a statistically significant difference is reported, the individual implications for therapy are often difficult to extrapolate or interpret. The statistical procedures employed in a large-N group-comparison study involve the comparison of average performance across groups of clients. Therefore, one cannot readily extrapolate the findings to any individual client. Hersen and Barlow (1976, p. 16) state that when the large-N group-comparison method is used, ''some patients will improve and others will not. The average response, however, will not represent the performance of any individual in the group.'' In the traditional group-comparison approach, regardless of the significance level, the particular clients who receive treatment and who benefit from it cannot be distinguished from those clients who also receive the intervention but who benefit by chance. Statistical significance as described previously is necessarily viewed in terms of an average over a wide range of individuals and their characteristics (IQ, sex, age, etc.), and the greater the heterogeneity of the sample, the less the data indicate for which values of the parameters in the sample the treatment effect was real.

The clinical implications of the inability to extrapolate findings from group-comparison designs to specific clients in particular clinical settings should be obvious. As Strupp and Bergin (1969, p. 11) note, clinicians need to know "what treatment, by whom, is most effective for this individual, with that specific problem, and under which set of circumstances."

Another limitation of group-comparison research designs in clinical settings is related to the ability or inability to generalize the findings to a larger target population. As discussed previously, the purpose of selecting and observing a sample is to make inferences from the sample to the parent or target population (or distribution). The validity of such inferences depends on the randomness of the sample in relation to the target population. Suppose that the subjects chosen for a group-comparison design are actually selected by some appropriate method of randomization (with such devices as stratifying and pairing allowed for) from an existing, well-defined group of clients who are representative of a large target population. Then there can be little question concerning the applicability or extension of inferences drawn from a statistical analysis of the data beyond the sample clients to other clients representing the larger target population. Such a model is well established in the deductive, theory-testing, group-comparison research approaches widely employed and advocated in the behavioral and social sciences. For example, suppose that the data from a randomly selected sample show a statistically significant difference favoring treatment A over treatment B for some disorder. Then a decision in favor of treatment A is clearly indicated for intervention in other clients with the same disorder who have been randomly selected from the target population. Replications of this finding add considerable strength to this decision and the theoretical position that supports it. This, of course, follows from the expectation, based on the design model, that on average a greater percentage of similar clients would improve with treatment A than with treatment B.

Now, if we consider an obvious practical limitation of clinical research design, we often find that the same difficulties which are involved in obtaining a well-balanced, group-comparison design with a sufficiently large number of clients are also encountered in extending statistical results to a larger target population. If, within a clinical environment, all available clients who meet a set of criteria for a study need to be selected to obtain a reasonable sample, there can be few, if any, clients left who meet the same criteria and who therefore can be considered as representative of the target population in a strictly statistical sense. Consequently, one has few clients left for a statistically valid application of the significant findings of the group-comparison design. At best, under the limitations described above, it is fairly evident that the population of reference corresponding to the group-comparison design model in clinical settings is often very limited.

The group-comparison approach also presents problems when it is used prematurely or inappropriately, particularly in clinical settings. True differences between groups may be obscured by a number of factors, alone or in combination. Among these factors are the quality of the measuring device, uncontrolled or unknown background or secondary variables, and small sample size. For instance, the more imprecise a measuring instrument is, the more error or variance is introduced into the observations. Differences observed in performance between groups would have to be large (large treatment effect) to override the gross measures of performance. This is particularly true for small samples, as alluded to earlier.

Finally, a lack of control of background characteristics of the clients being compared not only may obscure differences but also may confound the interpretation of results when a significant difference does occur. The more heterogeneous the sample, the more difficult the designation of which variables were responsible for the significant changes that were observed. Human behavior is complex, and a large number of secondary variables may contribute to changes or improvements in performance. In traditional group-comparison designs employed in clinical settings, it is often impossible to control or account for the effect of multiple background variables across heterogeneous samples.

CONCLUSION

In spite of the limitations described previously, large-N group-comparison designs remain extremely potent and useful methods of research investigation when the requirements to adequately implement them can be met. These types of designs are well established in behavioral and social science research and have provided valuable information related to the development and testing of various theoretical predictions. The point that is emphasized here and elaborated on throughout the remaining chapters is that group-comparison designs are not appropriate or practical for use in many clinical situations. Although group-comparisons of data provide valuable information related to group performance, the practitioner is more likely to be interested in information relevant to the ability of individual clients. Obviously, there is a need for research strategies and designs that will provide both types of information. Traditionally, research and evaluation in field and clinical settings have been associated with group-comparison designs. These methods often have weaknesses that limit their usefulness in applied or clinical environments. Fortunately, alternative strategies more compatible with the demands of clinical environments are available. Unfortunately, these methods are not widely understood or employed by practitioners who could benefit most from their adoption. In

Chapter 3, the general characteristics of single system research and evaluation methods are presented. The advantages of these procedures in demonstrating client change and therapist accountability are explored in more detail. Single system methods are briefly compared and contrasted with more traditional group-comparison procedures, and the argument is made that single system designs are better suited to monitor practice and evaluate individual client change related to treatment in clinical settings, while group-comparison methods are more appropriate for establishing the validity of theoretical positions that are used as general guides for clinical practice.

CHAPTER 3

Introduction to Single System Evaluation Strategies

INTRODUCTION

Within the fields of occupational and physical therapy, there is an increasing demand from both consumers and professionals for clinical practitioners to be accountable for the outcomes of the therapeutic strategies that they employ in the delivery of services to clients and patients with handicapping conditions (Gillette, 1982; Payton, 1979). As alluded to in previous chapters, this is a healthy demand, as it reflects the rehabilitation community's optimism that socially valued outcomes for therapeutic procedures used by occupational and physical therapists are obtainable. Based on the developing empirical literature, such an optimism appears to be justified. Such an optimism, however, cannot be said to be reflected in the actual day-to-day practice in many physical and occupational therapy clinics and related practice environments. The lack of transfer or integration of rehabilitation research findings to clinical settings is discouraging. Much of what therapists practice and how they practice it continues to be based on conjecture and anecdotal evidence or, at best, on a theory that has logical or personal appeal and traditional acceptance. These practices produce a time-honored, if not empirically supported, therapy system. For the outcomes of empirical research to become part of a powerful therapeutic technology, research outcomes must be integrated with field or clinical application. For this to become a reality, research findings must be presented to therapists, preferably in their early training, in such a manner that they can, and will, use them in clinical practice. In addition, therapists must acquire specific skills in research methodology so that they can critically examine current research literature and actively fulfill their own role in the evaluation of a therapeutic technology by validating and integrating clinical research findings in their clinical settings.

At present, therapists and other practitioners in the health-related services tend to emerge from their education and training with the belief that research is far removed from their professional needs and with little realization that they can play an active role in contributing to the advancement of an empirically based therapeutic practice. The courses in research methodology available to undergraduate or postgraduate students in the therapy disciplines appear to be based on traditional large-N group-comparison research procedures, and this may be one important reason for the lack of integration of research and practice to any appreciable degree. Courses or textbooks emphasizing single system designs or small-N research in the rehabilitation fields are conspicuous by their absence.

Although much valuable therapeutic knowledge can be gained through the use of group-comparison research methods, such procedures present fundamental difficulties for those working with clients in applied or clinical settings. As noted in Chapter 2, this is particularly true for the clinician working with the low-instance populations that are often encountered in clinical environments. As also noted in Chapter 2, group-comparison approaches rely on statistical inferences from averaged group data. Responses of individuals within the group, which may vary widely, are therefore not assessed; as a result, it is difficult to make reliable therapeutic decisions concerning the effective intervention strategies for specific clients. Other limitations include (1) the ethical problem of withholding treatment from a no-treatment control group, (2) the difficulty of locating large homogeneous groups of clients with similar disorders, (3) the cost in terms of funding and the time required to acquire large groups, as well as to collect and analyze the data, and (4) the reliance on statistically significant findings to make effectiveness decisions, as opposed to the therapeutically significant results required of clinical research.

Due to these and other limitations discussed previously, the argument has been made that single system designs offer a viable alternative to group-comparison research for those working in clinical settings (Bloom and Fischer, 1982; Kazdin, 1982). An examination of the wealth of experimental single-case research conducted by applied researchers in other fields, such as clinical psychology and special education, over the past several years certainly adds weight to this viewpoint. Without specific training in evaluation research procedures based on individual performance, however, it appears unlikely that occupational or physical therapists will develop the competence to evaluate the results of small-N research methodology, much less to integrate such research methods into their own clinical practices.

The purpose of this chapter is to provide an overview of the main strategies and issues related to single system procedures in the context of their relevance to occupational and physical therapy practice. Subsequent chapters provide more detailed material related to many of the designs and issues introduced in this section.

COMPONENTS OF SINGLE SYSTEM _____ EVALUATION AND RESEARCH _____

Single system designs basically involve studying a single individual or system (group) by taking repeated measurements of one or more dependent variables and systematically applying and, sometimes, withdrawing or varying the independent variable. If the application, withdrawal or manipulation of the treatment is associated with systematic changes in the dependent variable, it is inferred that the treatment has produced the changes.

Bloom and Fischer (1982) introduced the term single system design to refer to the repeated collection of information on a single system over time. They define the system as ''an individual, family, group, organization or other collectivity'' and note that for analysis purposes each is treated as a single unit. Bloom and Fischer (1982) contend that the term single system is more flexible and representative than some of the more traditional labels such as single-subject, single-case, small-N, time-series, or idiographic research. Regardless of the terminology employed, all single system designs discussed in later chapters have at least two features in common. The two major components of single system designs are (1) the sequential application and withdrawal or variation of the intervention and (2) the use of frequent and repeated outcome measures.

Sequential Application, Withdrawal, or Variation of Treatment

A single application of a treatment is generally not considered sufficient to establish an association of cause and effect. Rather, the emphasis in single system designs is on the sequential application, withdrawal, or variation of the intervention. A unique feature of single system designs is that they provide a comparison for intervention during the baseline. The baseline consists of the systematic collection of data on the problem prior to the actual introduction of intervention. The data collected during the baseline are used to help establish a pretreatment rate of performance that is used as a basis of comparison after the treatment is introduced and additional data are collected. The data collected during the actual intervention phase are compared with performance that occurred during the earlier baseline phase. The letter A is traditionally used to signify the baseline phase. Baseline data are generally collected until a stable response pattern is established. This may mean collecting baseline data for variable periods, from hours to days to a couple of weeks. Sometimes, a stable baseline may be impossible to obtain. When a stable level of pretreatment performance cannot be obtained, various statistical techniques may be employed to smooth out the unstable response pattern. These techniques are presented in more detail in Chapter 8.

Following the collection of baseline information, the intervention or treatment is introduced. In the simplest single system design, the treatment is generally referred to by the letter B. During the intervention phase, the therapist continues to record information on the client's performance in the same manner used during the baseline period. Obviously, the therapist is hoping to see a change in client performance when the treatment is introduced in the B phase. There may be as many A and B phases as is feasible or necessary to establish clear control over the dependent measure by the treatment (see Figure 3.1). For this study to be distinguished from a simple case study in which a subject's characteristics and performance are described, often in an anecdotal fashion, there must be some manipulation of the intervention, i.e., an introduction, withdrawal, or variation of the treatment.

Generally, it is advisable in most single system designs to have at least two applications and withdrawals of the independent variable or intervention. This is due to the possible confounding effects of history if an initial baseline period is followed by only one application and withdrawal of a program or treatment. For example, if a client who is involved in a therapeutic exercise program begins to demonstrate a loss of weight and a drop in blood pressure, we would like to infer that this result was "caused" by the introduction of a home exercise program developed because the client was at high risk for a possible cerebrovascular accident (CVA). The AB design, however, doesn't exclude the fact that there may have also been a concurrent change in the client's diet that may have had something to do with the loss of weight and reduction in blood pressure. The AB design can clearly reveal if there has been a change in the dependent measure; the AB design, however, does not allow the therapist to rule out other possible "causes" for a change in behavior or performance that occurred coincidentally at the time that the treatment was introduced.

Repeated applications and withdrawals or variations of the intervention increase the therapist's confidence that chance events will not be matched coincidentally with each manipulation of the treatment. Hence, as the number of applications and withdrawals associated with changes in client performance increases, the confidence with which one can make inferences

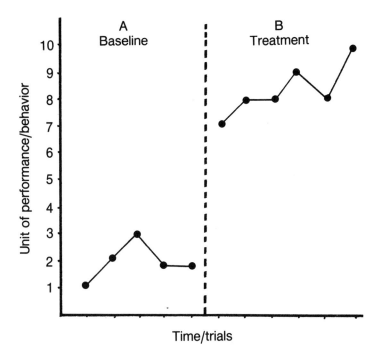

Figure 3.1. An example of an AB design showing response patterns for baseline and treatment phases.

about program effects also increases. We have more to say about design variations and the manipulation of intervention in later chapters in which specific design strategies employed in single system evaluation are discussed.

Frequent and Repeated Measures

The second major characteristic of single system designs that is associated with treatment evaluation and treatment research is the emphasis on repeated and frequent measurement of the dependent variable. In traditional group-comparison designs, the dependent variable is rarely measured more than twice (e.g., a pretest and a posttest). Measures are then averaged to obtain a mean score which is then compared across groups. In actual clinical situations, significant fluctuations in behavior or performance may occur at any time during the course of intervention, and repeated measures must be obtained during all phases of the design in order to investigate the cause of these fluctuations. This means that the outcome measures must be monitored frequently during the intervention phase as well as during the baseline periods. In addition, the use of pooled statistics that average data points within a particular phase is discouraged, since such averaging may obscure trends in the behavior being measured. The use of frequent and repeated measures allows the therapist to track individual performance on a continuous basis and to make modifications in the treatment as indicated.

A critical issue related to the use of repeated measures is the frequency of data collection. Special care must be taken to ensure that data are collected frequently enough to be able to match manipulations of the intervention with fluctuations in the outcome measures. Outcome measures, however, should not be taken so frequently as to fatigue or annoy the client. It is not possible to generate a firm set of rules regarding the optimal frequency for collecting outcome measures, since this will vary from measure to measure. Nevertheless, in general, as the natural or baseline variability in an outcome measure increases, the frequency of the collection of that measure should also increase. For example, if a particular outcome measure has large daily fluctuations, it should probably be monitored on at least a daily basis. On the other hand, an outcome measure that is fairly stable over weekly periods may be collected less frequently, once or twice a week would likely be sufficient. Sometimes, it is advisable for a therapist who is using a single system design to monitor prospective outcome measures in a pilot baseline phase to determine the natural variability of a particular outcome measure. This monitoring may be of particular help if the therapist is using a new outcome measure that has not previously been employed in the clinical setting. Those measures exhibiting a high degree of natural variability should subsequently be monitored more frequently than those with less natural variability.

Often, in a clinical environment, a treatment cannot be easily manipulated or withdrawn because of ethical considerations, lack of staff cooperation, or carryover effects (Barlow and Hersen, 1984). The presence of carryover effects may result in particular difficulty when some forms of single system design are applied to treatment evaluation, since treatment may produce changes in aspects of the client's performance or behavior which do not readily return to pretreatment levels when the intervention is withdrawn. For example, in the evaluation of the effectiveness of a program of therapy based on neurodevelopmental treatment (NDT) principles to improve the ambulation of a client who has suffered a CVA, it may be unreasonable to expect any improvement or increase in ambulatory skills to disappear when the treatment is withdrawn. For such a case the power of an ABA design may be weak, since a withdrawal of therapy would not be expected to result in a return to preintervention baseline performance. Consequently, other forms of single system design have been developed for use when the effects of the intervention cannot be reversed or withdrawn.

These designs are presented in more detail in later chapters, and only the multiple baseline design is introduced here.

Multiple baseline designs involve application of the same independent variable in a randomly determined sequence to separate, it is hoped, (1) independent behaviors in a given client, (2) the same behavior across different clients, or (3) a single client or group of clients across independent settings. In this design, the still-untreated baseline serves as a control for the previously treated behaviors, subjects or settings (see Figure 3.2). One can infer program effects only if application of the independent variable to one behavior, subject, or setting is associated with changes in the outcome measure for that behavior, subject, or setting and not with changes in any of the untreated baselines. This inference is strengthened each time the finding is replicated, as the treatment is sequentially applied to each of the behaviors, subjects, or settings.

An illustration of a multiple baseline design across three subjects is shown in Figure 3.2. In this illustration, the program is first applied to client 1 (subject 1), while it is withheld from clients 2 and 3 (subjects 2 and 3). The dependent measure, however, is monitored for all three subjects. Subsequently, the treatment is introduced to the second client and finally to the third client. In this illustration, one is able to infer treatment effects, since changes in the dependent measure occurred in each client's performance only after the intervention was implemented for that client.

When it is not possible to withdraw the independent variable, multiple baseline designs and their variations provide an alternate way to evaluate the influence of the program being used. Multiple baseline designs are particularly appealing to therapists and appear frequently in the applied behavioral analysis literature. An added attraction of the multiple baseline design is the built-in replication which strengthens the inferences that may be drawn from the design. The multiple baseline design and several related variations are presented in Chapter 6.

Internal Validity and Single System Designs

The use of frequent measures in single systems designs introduces two potential confounds, namely, testing and instrumentation. As noted in Chapter 2, testing may be a threat to the internal validity of a study when the behavior of an individual or group is altered simply by the process of monitoring or measuring that behavior. This would appear to be a particularly troublesome problem, because reactivity to the measurement may be more pronounced with single system designs than with designs in which measurements are only taken at two points (pretest and posttest). Indeed, with single system designs, there is a potential for testing effects to interact with treatment phases. For example, following collection of baseline data,

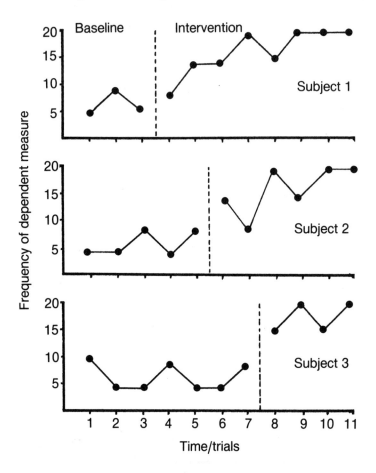

Figure 3.2.   An example of a multiple baseline design across subjects.

a group of institutionalized mentally retarded residents is provided a program of weight-reducing exercises. When the program is withdrawn in the second A phase of an ABA design, the continued monitoring of the individual participants' weights may inspire them to continue weight reduction activities on their own because of what they learned during the intervention phase. If this happens, the therapist who is conducting the evaluation may falsely conclude that decreases in weight were due to some historical event not related to the intervention, rather than to the treatment program itself. Conversely, continued monitoring during the withdrawal phase might demoralize the residents by reminding them that they have lost the benefits of the programmed activities. In the latter instance, the effects of the intervention might appear to be greater than they actually were.

In view of the drawbacks related to frequent or repeated measurement, it seems advisable for the therapist employing single system designs to try and use unobtrusive or nonreactive outcome measures whenever possible. Depending on the nature of the treatment and the type of performance being evaluated, it may be possible to obtain measurements covertly. This would help to reduce the reactivity of the measurement procedure. Covert observation and recording of client performance, however, are generally not options available in most clinical settings. It should be emphasized that if measurements are conducted on a regular basis throughout the evaluation, any reactive effects related to observation would be distributed evenly across all phases of the evaluation. In other words, the effects would be manifest in both the intervention and the nonintervention period. The argument could still be made that the reactivity due to repeated measurements was responsible for some patient improvement and would obscure the actual magnitude of the treatment. Thus, the treatment could appear more effective than it really was. We have more to say about measurement techniques in Chapter 4. For a more thorough discussion of nonreactive measurement procedures, the interested reader may consult Kazdin (1979) or Webb et al. (1981).

Instrumentation effects also may confound single system designs. Instrumentation becomes a threat when changes in the outcome measure are due to alterations in the instrument used to collect the dependent measure, rather than to manipulation of the intervention. Since single system designs involve the repeated collection of data at different times, it seems particularly important to ensure that systematic changes in the methods of collecting the outcome measures do not occur. One safeguard against confounding treatment effects with instrumentation is to include multiple applications and withdrawals of the intervention, which thus makes it less likely that systematic changes in the method of data collection will coincide precisely with the manipulation of the independent variable. In addition, prior to the evaluation, particular care should be taken to develop fully the outcome measures to be used in the program evaluation, and frequent reliability checks should be made to ensure that the method of data collection remains relatively constant throughout the assessment period (Johnston and Pennypacker, 1980; Kazdin, 1982).

As noted earlier in this chapter, history can also be a threat to internal validity of single system designs if changes in the dependent measure are due to historical events rather than to program effects. With the ABA reversal design, a historical event may, by chance, be associated with one introduction or withdrawal of the independent variable; it is highly unlikely, however, that such a historical event would consistently be associated with every application and withdrawal of the independent variable. With the multiple baseline design, assessing the possible effects of historical events is somewhat more complicated. In the simplest case, a historical event would show changes both in the treated client, the behavior, or the setting and in the untreated baselines. As pointed out earlier, if this occurred, one could not infer that the changes were due to the application of the treatment. It is conceivable, however, that treated and untreated clients may be differentially responsive to the occurrence of a given historical event, because of the possible nonequivalence of the clients. In this case, observed changes in the treated clients may be due to either the treatment effects or the influence of history. Thus, when multiple baseline designs are used, it is vital that causal specification be withheld, pending subsequent application of the treatment and observation of treatment effects in previously untreated clients, behaviors, or settings. Given that replication of the treatment effects can be adequately demonstrated, however, the multiple baseline design also offers adequate control over historical influences.

In general, those threats that are controlled for by random assignment to groups in traditional group-comparison designs are similarly controlled for in single system designs by the multiple application and variation or withdrawal of the intervention and by the use of repeated measures. As noted in Chapter 2, random assignment is generally considered the most powerful method of controlling for threats to internal validity in traditional group-comparison designs. The probability that random assignment of clients to treatment and control groups will actually distribute all possible confounds equally across the two groups is, however, a function of both the number of subjects available for assignment and the homogeneity of the sample. The argument was previously made that in most clinical settings the small number of clients available and the heterogeneity of the clients would seriously weaken the effectiveness of random assignment to minimize threats to internal validity. Even if optimal conditions did exist in a particular evaluation effort, and random assignment was employed, it is still important for the therapist to realize that potentially confounding factors are not eliminated or even identified by the use of random assignment. The effects of possible confounds are simply distributed across conditions in a fashion that is not likely to result in bias favoring one group over another.

White (1984, p. 116) has stated that, given the practical limitations of controlling the various threats to internal validity in clinical research by use of traditional group-comparison procedures,

single-case evaluations are also likely to prove more satisfactory in the demonstration of internal validity. While most of the same threats to internal validity exist for both the group and single-case evaluation design, the group statistical approach usually seeks to control for those threats by distributing potential confounding factors evenly among the various evaluation groups. The single-case approach obviates one of the most serious threats to internal validity (biased sample selection) and allows for the direct observation of other threats.

As noted earlier, the use of repeated measures does require that the therapist who uses single system designs be especially aware of the possible confounding influences of testing and instrumentation effects. The use of nonreactive and reliable forms of measurements, in addition to the sequential application and withdrawal of the treatment, appears to provide adequate control over these two threats to internal validity, however (Kazdin, 1982; Kratochwill, 1978). In multiple baseline strategies, threats to internal validity related to assessment are controlled for by the comparison of the treated behaviors, subjects, or settings with the untreated baselines.

In addition to their capability to monitor or control for the majority of those threats which are normally controlled for in group-comparison designs by random assignment (see Robinson and Foster, 1979), single system designs are better able to minimize many of the threats (identified by Cook and Campbell (1979)) to internal validity for *field* experiments. This is because in a single system design, all of the clients receive the program. Hence, there is little possibility of one group of clients feeling ''left out'' or of administrative contamination of an evaluation by providing the control group with some different intervention.

There is, however, the introduction of a new problem. Although differential reactions across clients may be minimized with single system designs, reaction effects within a subject become more suspect. That is, if a client alternately receives a treatment and then has the treatment withheld, he or she may begin to feel manipulated. A client may react negatively to such a perception or terminate participation in the program, which leaves an incomplete evaluation. In addition, therapists may be reluctant to withdraw a treatment which they feel is having a positive effect. In this respect, it seems that multiple baseline designs offer more control over within-subject reaction effects. One should note, however, that as the length of the initial baseline period in multiple baseline designs increases, the possibility of within-subject reaction effects also increases. The interested reader is referred to Kratochwill (1978) for a more detailed discussion of the issues of internal validity as they relate to single system designs.

External Validity and Single System Designs

Usually it is assumed that group-comparison designs in which subjects are randomly selected from a large target population are necessary to establish an acceptable degree of external validity. As noted in Chapter 2, however, some researchers using single system designs have argued that group-comparison designs often have limited generalizability. For maximum external validity it is assumed that the groups studied must be

representative of the target population. If all relevant population characteristics are indeed sampled, the group will be fairly heterogeneous. The
more heterogeneous the sample, the less the findings based on average
results will reflect any given individual's outcome. Therefore, if one
wishes to determine whether a particular treatment has a beneficial effect
for a *specific client*, a traditional group design is inadequate. Consequently,
proponents of single system designs advocate studying individual subjects
in the belief that only by emphasizing the variability inherent in all program
outcomes, and not by treating it as error that must be statistically controlled, can one begin to understand and reveal the complex relationship
between treatment and client outcomes.

The generality of findings from single subject methods is often discussed
in relation to between-group research. Because large numbers of subjects
are used in between-group designs compared with single system methods,
the findings are often assumed to be more generalizable. The use of large
numbers of subjects in a research design does not, of itself, ensure generalizability (Chassan, 1979; Sidman, 1960).

In the vast majority of between-group investigations, results are evaluated on the basis of average performance across groups. The use of analyses
based on pooled data does not shed light on the generality of the intervention effects among individuals. Indeed, in any particular between-group
investigation, there is the possibility that a statistically significant difference was obtained on the basis of chance (Type I error). The results may not
generalize to other attempts to replicate the study or to different categories
of subjects. In single system research, extended assessment across both
treatment and no-treatment (baseline) phases makes it implausible that any
intervention effects could be attributed to chance.

In relation to external validity, White (1984, p. 117) provides a cogent
argument for use of single system designs:

The replicated single-case approach has most often been attacked as incapable of
adequately assessing population validity, but the ability to do just that is probably its
strongest point. Since each student represents a self-contained evaluation of program
effects, every student involved in the overall study represents a meaningful replication
and provides direct evidence of the degree to which generalization across pupils might
be expected. The typical group-statistical design, on the other hand, is incapable of
assessing the significance of program impact at an individual level and must rely on
student selection strategies to build a "logical" case for generalizability of effect.
Indeed, since statements of individual effect are usually not possible in the group-
statistical design, such designs are generally incapable of assessing even the degree of
generalized effects within the evaluation sample itself, let alone to some broader
population.

Some other advocates of single system designs have also suggested that the results may be more generalizable than those obtained in between-group research because of the methodology and goals of these alternative approaches (cf. Baer, 1977). As Kazdin (1982) notes, the problem of single system research is not that the results lack generality among subjects. Rather, the problem is that there are difficulties largely inherent in the methodology for assessing the dimensions that may dictate generality of the results. Within single system research, there are no provisions for identifying subject-treatment interactions within a single patient. Focusing on one subject does not allow for the systematic comparison of different treatments among multiple subjects who differ in various characteristics, at least, within a single study.

Given that single system designs do not employ large numbers of randomly selected clients, how can the generality of a treatment's effectiveness be established with use of single system designs? Barlow and Hersen (1984) describe three phases involved in establishing the generalizability of single system evaluation research. The first phase involves the accumulation of a number of direct replications of the specific treatment effect on one well-defined dependent measure within a given clinical setting. During this phase, clients would be matched as closely as possible on all feasible subject variables. The aim is to establish, as clearly as possible, that a given intervention can have an effect on a certain kind of client within a specific setting. Obviously, the ability to generalize to other settings or human service providers would be limited.

The second phase involves the systematic replication of the program or treatment across various clients, settings, therapists, or any combination of these. Systematic replication helps to establish the generality of the findings over a wider range of situations than does direct replication.

The last phase of replication identified by Barlow and Hersen (1984) is clinical replication. Clinical replication involves establishing the generality of a treatment package that includes two or more procedures.

It is noteworthy that most evaluators employing single system designs would not generally advocate that all three of the above phases be carried out within one specific clinical situation. Rather, it would be argued that such extensive evaluations of programs would best be handled by a wide variety of clinicians and researchers. The reader is referred to Barlow and Hersen (1984) for more information on the issue of external validity in single system designs.

The topics of internal and external validity are discussed again in Chapter 9, after additional information on design and analysis procedures associated with single system strategies is presented.

Advantages of Single System Designs

In Chapter 2, several inherent difficulties and limitations of clinical designs based on the traditional group-comparison approach were detailed. The perception that group-comparison "true" experimental designs are the sine qua non of experimentally valid research is changing. For example, Cronbach (1982, pp. 29–30) recently noted:

> Those who press for rigor have always been ambivalent about quasi-experiments because the category includes both close and distant approximations. In fact, Campbell and Stanley [1963] overshot their mark. Aiming to show that careful interpretation could make good use of quasi-experiments, they inadvertently lead some less sophisticated readers to believe that quasi-experiments are suspect. Some readers were even persuaded that a design that classifies subjects into types before assigning them to treatment at random is inferior to a fully random assignment. Readers were also led to think of [true] experiments as impeccable, but the ideal experiment can rarely be achieved. A randomized design in a field study is likely to provide no more than an approximation to a true experiment, because of attrition and other departures from the plan.

Cronbach (1982, p. 57) in a later chapter notes that "convincing reasoning about causation, then, may be possible in almost any kind of design. Once more we see the limitations of a classification system that leads to appraisal, in the abstract, of some types of design as excellent and others as defective."

As noted previously, the basic unit of variability in traditional group-comparison designs is computed based on variation *between* clients, with means, percentages and variability relating to group performance. On the other hand, the basic unit of variability in single system designs is based on *within-subject* performance while the client's behavior is recorded repeatedly. Thus, a single system design for the purpose of evaluating the effect of a specific treatment with respect to a given client will consist of a series of intervention phases implemented over a period of time and the corresponding observations of individual client performance during those phases. Within the duration of such a design, there may be several introductions and reversals or withdrawals of the intervention. The recording of client performance is continuous throughout the period of evaluation.

Single system approaches to evaluating client performance are currently being widely advocated as an empirically legitimate alternative to more traditional group-comparison approaches, particularly in clinical environments in which group-comparison approaches are often of limited use (Bloom and Fischer, 1982; Kazdin, 1982). For example, Kazdin (1983, p. 424) recently noted that single system strategies "represent a scientific methodology that can evaluate alternative treatments and rule out the impact of extraneous factors as rival explanations of the results. More importantly, the methodology provides a flexible approach that is consistent with many of the priorities, professional responsibilities and practical exigencies of clinical practice.''

The primary advantage of a single system evaluation strategy is the ability of such an approach to identify characteristics relevant to client performance. If an experimental group of 50 clients does statistically better than a control group of 50 clients, such a difference could be due to a small number of clients in the treatment group showing large changes while the majority of clients in the treatment group show no change or perhaps even deteriorate slightly (Jayaratne and Levy, 1979). As noted previously, individual variations are masked by the group average. Furthermore, as Chassan (1979) points out, the group-statistical design does not permit conclusions as to which particular client characteristics correlate with improvement or deterioration. These data are lost in the statistical analysis. Findings, therefore, are not readily translatable to the practicing clinician. In the single system approach in which each client serves as his or her own control, effective treatments can be linked with specific client characteristics that are immediately relevant to the clinical therapist. Once a clinically significant difference appears within a single system design, the therapist can specify the particular client variables and other relevant factors present when the clinically significant result was obtained. In the single system approach, not only are such factors as sex, age, diagnosis, level of disability, and intelligence kept constant, but so also are all possible significant life experiences up to the beginning of the intervention. This degree of individual control is obviously not possible in the group-comparison model.

In a group-comparison design, a treatment ''works'' if it produces a statistically more significant effect than some control or comparison procedure. Although this type of finding is valuable in the testing of a specific theoretically derived hypothesis, such a finding may have limited clinical usefulness. With single system strategies, the size of the treatment effect is directly measured in individual clients, facilitating judgments of clinical utility.

The effectiveness of a given treatment in a traditional group-comparison design is usually assessed once just after the treatment is completed. This strategy precludes the continuous assessment and analysis of the client's course during treatment, which may vary from day to day. A single system design in which measures are continually gathered allows the therapist to observe variability and to relate environmental or personality variables to client performance. Designs based on the intensive study of the individual client allow more flexibility than is possible in traditional group-comparison methods. The accumulation of data on an on-going basis allows a systematic analysis of the course of treatment and may suggest useful modifications of the design as the study progresses. Within the framework of the single system design, the therapist can take into account and analyze the impact of day-to-day contingencies and related events that effect client behavior.

The use of single system designs to evaluate clinical practice also changes the evaluator's orientation toward the use and type of dependent measure that should be employed to assess clinical change. If one is oriented toward the use of group-comparison methods in which basic statistical tests and comparisons are made between groups of clients, it seems natural to develop measuring instruments that are sufficiently general to include the various examples of group "behavior" under a single word or term or, at best, under a few such terms for each behavior. The use of high-level or broad abstractions contributes to the measurement difficulties associated with evaluation and operationalization of client performance in traditional group-comparison approaches. Once the emphasis is placed on a single system approach, it is natural to develop measurement procedures specific to the individual. One can then stay close to the specific manifestations of a given client's behavior or performance in the construction of an outcome measure. For example, it would be much easier for two observers on a given day to agree on whether or not a client wears his shirt inside out than to agree on whether his behavior is "bizarre."

Single systems methods can be readily incorporated into routine clinical programming for each client without any significant disruption of the usual therapeutic routine. In addition, single system designs are essentially theory free and can be applied to evaluate the effectiveness of any therapeutic strategy regardless of theoretical orientation. The primary goal of single system methods is not to validate a theoretical position but to demonstrate the individual effectiveness of a particular intervention strategy. Bloom and Fischer (1982, p. 15) state:

They [these methods] provide a model for demonstrating our accountability to ourselves, our clients and consumers, our funding sources, and our communities. Systematic, consistent use of single system designs will allow practitioners, and agencies, to collect a body of data about the effectiveness of practice that provides more or less objective information about the success of our practice.

Single system designs fulfill several different functions related to treatment research and treatment evaluation in occupational and physical therapy. First, the absence of a clear research methodology or set of evaluation strategies designed for the individual client helps to exacerbate the functional hiatus between clinical research and clinical practice. In many of the helping and rehabilitation professions, there is often a split or poor connection between research and practice (Ballin et al., 1980; Hunt, 1981). Persons in applied fields who conduct traditional research rarely also engage in clinical practice, and persons engaged in clinical practice rarely also conduct traditional research (Strupp, 1981). Treatment research is often conducted in academic settings where the conditions of treatment administration and the type of clients may be quite different from those found in the average clinical setting. As a result, traditional empirical investigations often have little bearing on the questions and concerns of practitioners (Fishman, 1981). Treatment research typically evaluates one or more techniques presented to groups of subjects in a standardized fashion. Conclusions about treatment effectiveness are based on the average amount of change as evaluated by statistical significance. Therapists, on the other hand, are concerned with evaluating treatments applied to individuals and are interested in the capability of those treatments to produce clinically significant changes in the client's everyday function.

As noted previously, part of the problem is that traditional clinical research investigations are invariably conducted with groups of persons in order to meet the requirements of traditional group-comparison designs and statistical evaluation. Investigation of groups and conclusions based on pooled patient performance, however, can misrepresent the effects of treatments for specific individuals.

The practicing therapist is confronted daily with the individual client, and it is at this level that empirical evaluations of treatment need to be made. The problem, of course, is that the primary empirical tool available to the clinical therapist has, until recently, been the uncontrolled case study in which anecdotal information is reported and from which scientifically accepted inferences cannot be drawn (Bolgar, 1965; Yin, 1984). The single system designs presented throughout the remaining chapters of this text provide a systematic methodology to improve the information that can be drawn from individual clients. The designs permit therapists to identify and document systematic relationships in individual cases and, through accumulation of cases over a period of time, to identify general relationships that would otherwise be difficult or impossible to derive from uncontrolled case studies. Thus, single system designs can assist therapists in developing an empirically derived knowledge base for practice as well as for evaluation and documentation of the progress of individual clients.

Single system designs are ideally suited to address several important issues directly related to treatment evaluation with individual clients. The basic question for a therapist and client is whether a particular treatment is producing a therapeutic change. This question can be addressed by any one of several single system designs presented in the remaining chapters. In addition, certain designs allow comparisons of alternative treatments or of combinations of treatments for a given client. In treating individual clients, the therapist does not usually have the freedom or opportunity to apply a standardized treatment in a predetermined fashion or to assign subjects to treatment and no-treatment conditions. Rather, the therapist must try to produce therapeutic change and make decisions regarding treatment modifications in light of the client's performance. Single system designs permit changes important in improving or maintaining client progress to be made in the course of ongoing treatment. This is clearly an advantage with important implications for clinical evaluation and assessment.

The previous discussion is obviously biased in emphasizing the limitations of traditional group-comparison designs while highlighting the advantages of single system evaluation strategies. In reality, both approaches have identifiable strengths and weaknesses (see Table 3.1). The bias, however, was intentional. For many years, there has been an empirical prejudice favoring the use of group-comparison designs as the only legitimate form of ''research'' design. One objective of this text is to provide a viable clinical alternative to traditional group-comparison designs. A degree of initial ''bias'' will be required to help establish single system designs as clinically relevant and empirically respectable forms for evaluating treatment effectiveness.

Interest in single system methodology has rapidly increased in those disciplines, such as occupational and physical therapy, that have a major commitment to serving individual patients in an effective and efficient manner. Therapists are recognizing that single system strategies provide the ideal mechanism for conducting treatment evaluations. Several advantages of single system designs make the strategies particularly relevant for use by rehabilitation professionals. For instance, the designs can be used with low-incidence populations in which a variety of handicapping conditions are likely to exist. The designs are very flexible and can easily be adapted to fit the needs of a particular clinical setting or client. The designs emphasize the use of individualized measures of performance that are recorded on a regular basis throughout the evaluation period. This allows the analysis of the temporal pattern of client performance along with the final outcome and provides the therapist with a more accurate picture of total client function.

Single system methods are specifically designed to reveal individual differences and variability in performance, when these exist, and to allow the therapist to isolate variables directly contributing to changes in performance. Once these variables are isolated, they can be evaluated and, eventually, incorporated into the formal treatment program. The logic associated with single system designs is that individual variability should not be treated as error and eliminated but that such variability is a key component in the intervention process. Effective treatment programs can be developed only after the factors responsible for variation in individual

Table 3.1.

Comparison of Single System and Group-Comparison Research Approaches[a]

Single System Designs	Group-Comparison Designs
Involve only a single individual or a small group of subjects.	Involve at least two groups that are selected from a larger target population.
Responses to intervention are recorded repeatedly over a period of time. Responses are generally collected at regular intervals.	Responses are collected infrequently. They are often recorded prior to the introduction of intervention and again when the intervention is stopped.
Client feedback is carefully monitored as response data are collected, and, based on client feedback, the design phases may be modified. Process as well as outcome is studied.	Little or no data on client feedback are collected until the study is completed. The emphasis is on outcome, and little information is gathered relating to process.
Modifications in the design strategy are permitted. The methodology and measurement procedures are flexible.	The design is fixed, and changes in design strategy are not allowed once the intervention is introduced. Measurements are usually "standardized" and relatively inflexible.
The findings are directly or immediately relevant to a particular client. The results may not be readily generalizable to other clients.	Findings may be relevant to a particular "class" of subjects but are difficult to interpret for the individual.
The emphasis is on knowledge for immediate practical use, with secondary emphasis on knowledge building or theory testing.	The emphasis is on theory verification and hypothesis testing, with secondary emphasis on practical or immediate application.
Costs are relatively small, and the procedures can generally be incorporated as part of a clinical routine.	Costs are relatively high, and the procedures are difficult to implement in clinical settings without some outside resources or support.
The methods and procedures are relatively new, and statistical and inferential limitations are not completely understood.	Methods and procedures are well established and accepted as scientifically legitimate. Rules for statistical inference and generalizability are clearly defined.
Rely on variation *within* the individual to make judgments regarding the performance of a single subject or a small group.	Rely on variation *between* individuals to make inferences about group performance.

[a]Adapted from: Ottenbacher, K. (1984). Nomothetic and idiographic strategies for clinical research: in apposition or opposition. *Occup. Ther. J. Res., 4,* 198–212.

performance can be identified and examined in relation to treatment. White (1984) has accurately observed that single system strategies not only provide an alternative to more traditional methods but that they are probably the method of choice in the vast majority of situations in which health care professionals are attempting to evaluate therapeutic change.

CONCLUSION

This chapter outlines some of the characteristics and procedures that make single system designs different from those generally associated with "experimental" research. In review, there are two primary functions of single system strategies, as opposed to other more traditional methods. The first function is to monitor behavior or performance on an individual basis to determine whether or not a clinically important change has occurred. This is the primary function—a systematic comparison of baseline and intervention periods. Because this comparison does not require a sophisticated design, it is feasible to determine whether such changes occur with virtually all types of single system designs discussed in subsequent sections, including the most basic design, the AB design, which is introduced in this chapter.

The second function of single system evaluation strategies is to attempt to isolate the effects of a specific intervention and to determine the possible causal relationship between the intervention and any observed change in client performance or behavior. To make any causal inferences regarding whether a particular program of intervention resulted in or produced a change in client performance, the therapist generally needs a design that is more "powerful" than the basic AB design. The AB design is not able to rule out a number of other events that may have affected the client's behavior or performance during the intervention period. A number of more sophisticated or powerful single system designs are discussed in later chapters. These designs can reduce alternative explanations for changes in client performance and thereby increase our confidence in making causal inferences. As the sophistication of the designs increases, however, so does the difficulty of implementing them in a clinical environment without interrupting the regular clinical or therapeutic routine. Although these more complex designs strengthen the basis for drawing causal inferences between intervention and changes in client performance, it is also generally more difficult to apply these sophisticated single system designs in natural practice settings. In such settings, the basic AB design should be used as the minimal attempt at systematic evaluation. On the other hand, it is important to have a basic understanding of the design characteristics associated with more sophisticated single system designs. A therapist possessing this knowledge will be able to understand the use of such designs when they are encountered in the professional literature. In addition, when the opportunity to apply a sophisticated single system design presents itself, the therapist will be able to do so in an appropriate manner and will then be in a position to make more confident statements about causality in relation to the effectiveness of a particular intervention. Finally, familiarity with the basic principles of single system evaluation strategies will help the clinical therapist to become the scholarly practitioner demanded by the rehabilitation community and expected by consumers.

CHAPTER 4

Measurement and Recording Procedures Associated with Single System Designs

INTRODUCTION

The importance of observing, measuring and recording client performance or behavior is alluded to in Chapter 1. Accurate measuring and recording of behavior are necessary (1) to monitor the exact behavior that one desires to change and (2) to establish a baseline level of performance before a treatment procedure is implemented. During the course of intervention it is necessary to maintain an accurate system of measuring and recording behavior, so that treatment effects can be analyzed.

The significance of observation, measurement and recording procedures is not always recognized by therapists, nor are systematic procedures consistently used in most clinical environments. Some therapists reject the use of objective observational or recording techniques on the grounds that they are administrative or bureaucratic red tape. Such procedures are not considered a necessary or integral part of the therapeutic intervention process. As Bijou (1966) has argued, however, accurate observation and recording of behavior or performance indicates whether treatment procedures are effective and when they should be altered. If accurate recording strategies are maintained, it will no longer be necessary for the therapist to rely on "testimonial" statements about the efficacy of the intervention employed. Objective and accurate records will clearly demonstrate the merits of therapeutic intervention.

SPECIFYING THE BEHAVIOR AND/OR ——— PERFORMANCE TO BE MEASURED———

The first step in developing a strategy to accurately measure and record client change is to precisely define the behavior that is to be modified. All too often the performance which is the object of therapeutic intervention is couched in vague descriptions and explanations. For example, the following statement is a paraphrase of the ideas often encountered in texts for rehabilitation specialists:

The role of rehabilitation is to facilitate the healing and learning processes so that the maximum potential of every client or patient is realized. Therapy must enhance the physical and psychological performance and develop the unique abilities of each client or patient so that he or she can function as independently as possible.

Certainly this statement describes desirable, even ideal, therapeutic goals. "Maximum potential" and "unique abilities" are, however, vague terms which defy systematic measurement when they are applied to an individual patient. As a result, it may be difficult to know when an individual has achieved the objectives of rehabilitation. Also, because the procedures or techniques that "facilitate" the healing and learning process are not clearly specified, the means of achieving the objectives remain mostly unknown.

As Herbert and Attridge (1975, p. 7) point out, "all terms, especially those which designate items of behavior to be observed, must be as clearly and unambiguously defined as the behaviors under study will permit." Explicit definitions provide the basis for replicating the methods. Any effective or useful therapeutic program must be replicable. Replication must be possible not only within a specific clinical environment but also across clinical settings. Providing clear definitions is the first step in assuring that a therapeutic program will be replicable.

A clear definition is one that is easily read and unambiguous. It is consistent with the goals of treatment and is not easily confused with different or related behaviors. Thus, a clear definition can be readily paraphrased by others who can explain how the defined response differs from other behaviors.

An example of the care that should be exercised in defining the behavior to be altered by treatment is presented by Goodisman (1982). He conducted a study designed to investigate the effects of four distinct interventions on the ambulatory ability of a 5-year-old child with spastic dysplasia. Goodisman (1982, p. 285) states:

> Performance was measured by having the patient make three trips walking up and down a corridor each evening as close to 6 pm as possible. The patient was not told that he was being measured, nor was he told that anything special was expected of him. Nothing was indicated that would lead him to suspect the nature of the assessment going on.
>
> While the patient walked down the corridor, ''walking faults'' were counted and recorded by the primary observer. These were defined as characteristic steps that could lead to, or be associated with, balance instability. Five types of faults were recorded: dragging of the great toe, crossing one leg in front of the other, wandering of one leg away from the other, touching the corridor wall, and falling down.

In defining a specific target behavior, Johnston and Pennypacker (1980) have argued that the definition may be topographical or functional in nature. A topographical definition is one that emphasizes the movements or motor responses comprising a specific behavior or performance event. Sobsey and Orelove (1984) provide topographical definitions of various feeding behaviors in their study of eating skills in children with severe handicaps. They used a single system design to evaluate the effectiveness of various neurophysiological facilitation techniques to improve lip closure and rotary chewing in four severely handicapped children. Sobsey and Orelove (1984, p. 99) state that ''lip closure was recorded whenever the students' upper lip touched the spoon, food on the spoon, or the lower lip at midline.'' This description is topographical in nature, since it clearly emphasizes the movements that constitute the target behavior.

Functional definitions, according to Johnston and Pennypacker (1980), are those that emphasize the consequences of the behavior rather than its movement components. For instance, self-injurious behavior may be defined as any act that results in physical injury to the self. Hawkins (1982) contends that definitions that are functional provide the therapist with more useful information than do topographical definitions that stress movement components of behavior or performance. Functional definitions, however, tend to be more subjective and to be based more on assumptions and judgments made by the observer.

Once a behavior has been accurately defined, it can more easily be measured. All observable behaviors can be quantified in some manner by counting, timing or some combined measurement method. An empirical definition for a behavior should be worded so that the observable characteristics are clearly specified. If the behavior is properly defined, two or more observers or raters can then agree on the occurrence, frequency or duration of the behavior. Whatever constitutes an instance of behavior for one client must constitute an instance of behavior for another client. The behavior or event of therapeutic interest should be described so specifically that the occurrence of the behavior or event can be easily determined anytime any client displays the behavior (Cartwright and Cartwright, 1974).

If occupational and physical therapy are to function as legitimate rehabilitation professions and to base their practice on a scientific foundation, data on patient performance must conform to certain rigorous standards. Vague descriptors, nonfactual terms, or inner ''causes'' must be avoided when behaviors and performance outcomes are being defined. Therapeutic outcomes must not be stated too generally or arbitrarily if therapists are to accurately judge the occurrence or nonoccurrence of the behavior and the client's achievement of a useful therapeutic outcome. For example, terms such as improve or strengthen and goals such as reduce spasticity need further specification and are simply too vague to count, time, or measure systematically.

Definitional terms are functional guides for measurement only when they specify (1) observable or measurable action, activity, or movement which reflects the behavior of interest and (2) the behavior or event's onset or beginning and its ending. Additionally, the behavior or performance event identified for change should be discrete, so that it is repeatable.

A complete operational definition delineates the boundaries of the response so that in most situations an observer can discriminate it from other responses. Complete definitions should include the following: a descriptive name; a general operational definition; an elaboration of that definition, to point out how the response differs from other responses; and, ideally, some borderline or difficult examples of both the responses to be included and the responses to be excluded from the category. It is best to draw examples from actual events that can be observed in the treatment or the clinical setting where the recording will occur, so that they will be relevant. The examples should be accompanied by explanations of why they are to be included or excluded and of how the basic definition relates to the example.

Once the behavior which is to be the object of therapeutic intervention has been identified and succinctly defined, a method of observation and measurement of client performance may assume a wide variety of forms. Methods may vary with the behavior being measured.

STEPS IN OBSERVING AND RECORDING ———————————— BEHAVIOR ———————————

The six steps in the observation and recording of behavior are the following:

Step 1.   Determine the setting in which the behavior will be observed.
Step 2.   Decide on the method to be used to collect and code the behavior.
Step 3.   Decide the period of time that the behavior will be observed.
Step 4.   Observe and record client performance.
Sept 5.   Plot or record the data on a graph or chart.
Step 6.   Continue the procedures until the requirements of the overall design have been satisfied.

Step 1: Determine the Setting

In clinical environments the behavior or performance of therapeutic interest is generally related to a physical or psychological deficit. The dysfunction produces a reduced capacity or a maladaptive behavior. Ideally, the behavior should be observed in those situations in which it occurs naturally. For example, suppose an individual has severe rheumatoid arthritis and is unable to complete a simple activity of daily living (ADL) such as brushing his or her teeth. It would be desirable to observe and measure the behavior in the bathroom under the usual conditions surrounding or associated with tooth brushing.

The subject's natural environment has several advantages as the observational setting, most notably the fact that the therapist's goal is usually to understand or document the client's behavior in that environment, but it is not always the best situation in which to observe. In some "natural" settings, the frequency of the behavior may be too low or unpredictable. Observations can be unethical, or the observer's presence can be so intrusive that one can no longer refer to the environment as natural, as, for example, in the observation of some personal hygiene skills.

Occasionally, a therapist is able to combine observations in both a treatment setting and the natural environment. For example, Bonadonna (1981) investigated the effect of a program of vestibular stimulation on the incidence of stereotypic behavior in four severely mentally retarded persons. She (1981, p. 777) states that "the study was conducted at the subjects' school . . . [and that] two situations [were used] for data measurement: the experimental setting and the natural setting." The experimental setting in this study consisted of a 10- x 12-foot room containing selected pieces of equipment. The natural setting was defined as the child's regular classroom environment.

Step 2: Decide on a Method to Collect Data

The data must be collected and coded systematically. Several possible strategies are available for collecting data on the behavior of therapeutic interest. Four methods of collecting or recording data are in common use:

event recording, duration recording, rate recording, and time sampling (Altmann, 1974; Haynes, 1978).

Event Recording. In its simplest form, event recording consists of a simple tally of each occurrence of a defined response throughout an observation session. Tallying can be improved by recording the location of the observed responses in real time, which makes various forms of sequential and temporal analyses possible. Furthermore, a real-time record permits precise, event-by-event examination of agreements between more than one observer.

When the recorded behaviors only occur in discrete trials, the therapist may wish to record both the trial and the response. For example, the number of buttons correctly fastened by an arthritic client on a shirt with six buttons could be recorded. The client may be able to successfully button the three lowest buttons but be unable to button the top three buttons. The client would have successfully responded on 3 of the 6 trials.

Behaviors measured with use of event recording allow a therapist to count the number of times a particular behavior or performance event occurs in a specified, constant period of time. Event recording requires that the behavior be readily divided into countable, discrete units, with obvious beginning and termination points. Since the number of events provides a direct measure of the amount of behavior occurring, event recording is obviously sensitive to changes produced by intervention programs.

Event recording must be completed for equal units of time which are long enough to obtain a representative sample of the behavior. If the recording time cannot be uniform, the frequency of events cannot be used to evaluate performance, since they would not be comparable. For instance, the number of opportunities to perform in a 1-minute period is not equatable to those in a 30-minute period. In such a case, the frequency of events must be converted into rate per standard unit of time. Rate recording is described later in this chapter.

When a behavior occurs at a very high incidence or is ongoing and lasts for an extended period of time, an event recording procedure is generally inappropriate. In the former (behavior occurring very frequently), the probability of error is increased due to difficulty in counting. When behaviors of long duration are measured by use of an event recording procedure, the numerical result is deceiving. These data, reported as discrete events, will occur in such small amounts that changes in the behavior will not be detected. In such cases, duration recording provides a better description of a behavior than does event recording (Smith and Snell, 1978).

One additional kind of event recording should be noted: the interaction matrix recording described by Mash et al. (1976). In this method, a single mark indicates who within a dyad emitted what behavior and how the other person responded. The interaction matrix appears not to have gained wide clinical use, despite its promise as a tool for analysis of functional relations between interacting persons and its obvious relevance to therapeutic settings.

Duration Recording.   A duration record is needed when the focus is on the length of each occurrence of a response, on the time that it takes to complete a particular task, on the amount of time spent on a particular activity, or on the latency of a response. A duration record can be obtained by simply turning a stopwatch on and off. Electromechanical event recorders or electronic keyboards are commercially available and produce duration records while recording the onset and termination of other events. Duration recording may be used to determine the length of time that a child with cerebral palsy is able to maintain an erect head position or the amount of time it takes a cerebrovascular accident (CVA) client to eat a meal.

Duration of a behavior may be reported in terms of the total number of minutes (seconds, hours, etc.) or the percentage of time a behavior was engaged in during each observation period. Percentage reporting is especially useful if the observation sessions vary in length, since the resulting percentages are roughly comparable.

Duration recording, as does event recording, requires the complete and continuous attention of the observer during each period of observation. Duration records are most appropriate for behaviors or performance events when either have a high or an even rate or simply may be variable in their length from onset to end, which makes the frequency count a less meaningful measure.

Rate Recording.   Specifying the rate of behavior is a particularly popular method of recording client performance. Rate is generally defined as the frequency of a behavior divided by the time frame in which it occurred. For example, a behavior that occurred 10 times (frequency) within a 2-minute period (time frame) would have a rate of occurrence equal to 5 behaviors (sometimes referred to as movements) per minute. Rate of behavior as a measure of performance has a number of advantages. It reflects changes in either duration or frequency of response. It is a particularly sensitive measure for detecting changes or trends because it has no theoretical upper limit that could create an artificial ceiling effect. Although data based on rate recording reflect both duration and frequency, some authorities have argued that rate does not reflect either with acceptable accuracy (Altmann, 1974; Sackett, 1978).

Time Sampling.   Time sampling, which is also called scan sampling, instantaneous time sampling, discontinuous probe time sampling, and interval sampling, involves recording the state of a behavior at specific moments or intervals in time. These moments or intervals can be signaled to the recorder or observer by a simple kitchen timer, a cue recorded on an audio tape, or a pocket-size signal generator capable of emitting tones on a fixed or random schedule. As noted elsewhere (Hawkins, et al., 1976), time sampling is analogous to taking a still picture on each of many occasions and then inspecting each photograph to see whether a particular behavior was occurring. For example, therapists interested in determining the effect of an intervention program of specifically applied sensory stimulation on the incidence of self-abusive behavior in an autistic child might use a time sampling procedure. The therapist might observe the child for 5 seconds at 10-minute intervals for a 2-hour period each day. If during the 5-second period at the beginning of each 10-minute interval the child exhibits a self-abusive behavior, the therapist records this event. This example assumes that the behaviors to be classified as self-abusive have been previously defined.

With use of a time sampling strategy a therapist may record the number of responses occurring during a given interval. In such a case, a combination of time sampling and event recording would be used. Alternatively, the therapist may record the duration of a response during a given interval, in which case duration recording is combined with time sampling. Bonadonna (1981) employed this latter combination in the study referred to in a previous section. She (1981, p. 779) describes the recording strategy employed in her investigation:

Data were recorded using 30 second partial interval time samples. The first 30 seconds of a given minute were spent in observing the student's behavior and timing the duration of rocking behavior with a stopwatch. The second 30 seconds of that given minute were spent recording whether stereotypic rocking behavior occurred during the observation interval and total duration of rocking behavior for that interval. Every 30 seconds, "beeps" on a tape recorder noted whether it was an observation or recording interval . . . .

As with event and duration recording, the therapist's total attention must be directed toward the behavior during the interval of observation. In addition, with interval recording the observer must have some method of timing each interval so as to move from one interval to the next at the appropriate time. As noted previously, usually a stopwatch, kitchen timer, or the cue on a tape recorder is used.

The length of the interval for interval recording depends on the nature of the behavior (its length and frequency) and on the therapist's ability to record and attend. In the first case, the more frequent the behaviors, the smaller the interval for observation should be, so the observation may be an accurate measure of the behavior.

Repp et al. (1976) compared the accuracy of observations taken by various interval procedures to frequency measures of the same behavior for the same time period. Low and medium rates of responding were accurately measured with 10-second intervals, but high-rate response patterns, either of a continuously high rate or with sudden increases of high rates, were underestimated by interval measurements. Repp et al. (1976) recommend that intervals of less than 10 seconds be used to measure behaviors occurring at high response rates.

Regardless of the specific recording method used, therapists commonly tend to transform recorded behavior or events into percentage of "correct" responses. Percentages are straightforward and can be easily computed. There are, however, many ways in which percentages can be misleading, and therapists using correct responses recorded as a percentage should be aware of these limitations. For instance, percent correct scores do not provide any information about the actual number of times a client has performed correctly. For example, on Monday a client may complete an ADL task correctly 6 of 10 times, and on Tuesday the same client may perform the task correctly 3 of 4 times. The percentage correct for the two days are 60% and 75%, respectively. The increase does not mean that the client exhibited more correct responses on Tuesday; it only means that he or she made a higher proportion of correct responses. If the actual number of correct responses is important, the percentage statements can be misleading.

Another possible misinterpretation of percentage correct statements may occur if a different number of possible response times or trials are recorded during consecutive sessions. For instance, suppose lip closure is being evaluated in a client with oromotor dysfunction. On Monday, 10 trials are observed and the student demonstrates successful lip closure on 5 of the 10 trials. The student's percentage correct performance score is $5/10$ or 50%. On the next day, only 5 trials are allowed, but suppose that the client's performance ability has not changed. The client's response rate was 50% correct on the first day, which means that he or she was successful 5 of 10 times. If the client were 50% "correct" on the second day, he or she must successfully complete 2½ of the 5 trials. The client, however, cannot complete half of a trial successfully. If the behavioral units are simply and accurately defined, they should reflect an all-or-nothing performance. Either the client achieves lip closure (the target behavior) or the client does not. There are no half behavioral units. In other words, the client, who is provided only 5 trials on the second day, cannot demonstrate 50% accuracy. The client may complete 2 of the trials (40% correct performance) or 3 trials (60% correct performance). Compared with the first day's data, the second day's data would have to indicate that the client improved or got worse. A no-change statement or outcome is impossible because the percentage correct achieved on the first day cannot be achieved on the second day.

Recording performance in terms of percent correct response is not as simple or straightforward as it may appear initially. A therapist using this method of recording must be aware of its possible limitations so that misinterpretation of the data collected does not occur.

Step 3: Determine the Period of Time That Behavior Will Be Observed and Measured

Once a method of observing and measuring behavior has been devised, the next step is to determine the length of time necessary for obtaining baseline data and information related to the effects of treatment. Practices vary and no set interval of time for recording a baseline can be established that will be applicable to all settings. In general, baseline information should be collected until a stable pattern of responses emerges. Obtaining a stable response pattern prior to intervention will provide the foundation for making later comparisons with response patterns associated with treatment. A stable series of baseline observations will make the interpretation and analysis of data collected during the intervention periods much easier. The therapist should identify, depending on the nature of the behavior under study, a specific period of time which he or she estimates will be required to establish adequate baseline data. This period of time may range from hours to several days or weeks. The therapist should attempt to specify also the length of time each intervention phase will last. Again, this determination will depend on the nature of the problem or deficit under treatment, the type of intervention to be employed, and the setting and resources available to the therapist.

Step 4: Observe and Record Client Behavior

A baseline may be defined as the observation and recording of performance or behavior during the no treatment or nonintervention phase or phases. Baseline ratings should represent accurate measures of the client performance or behavior before treatment is initiated or at times when the treatment has been temporarily withdrawn. In a typical situation a baseline period will be followed by an intervention. During the treatment the behavior of therapeutic interest will continue to be measured in the same manner as was used during the baseline. Following a predetermined length of time the treatment may be temporarily terminated and a second baseline period may be introduced. If the second baseline period responses are the same or similar to the first, it may be assumed that the intervention produced any changes that were observed during the treatment phase. This approach may have some limitations in applied or clinical environments.

Obviously, once a certain treatment has produced a change, it may be undesirable to stop it, and even if it were terminated, the behavior may not return to the original baseline level. We have much more to say about baselines and related issues in the next two chapters dealing with specific single system design strategies.

Obviously, accurate recording of client responses during the baseline and intervention periods is essential, if reliable judgments are to be derived concerning client progress and the effectiveness of treatment. The initial step in gathering this data is to construct a data-recording form. Data-recording forms should be constructed to meet the following guidelines. First, the recording form must be compatible with the measurement procedure (e.g., event recording, duration recording). Second, the form must allow sufficient space to record data for each individual in a clear manner. The number of clients to be observed should be considered and their responses should be clearly separated and identified. Third, the form must accommodate the number of behaviors of therapeutic interest. The spaces for intervals or observation periods need to be appropriately subdivided and coded so that tallies or times recorded are identified with the behavior with which they are associated. Fourth, when event recording is used, enough space must be allowed for slash marks or other methods of marking. The more frequent the behavior, the more space that must be allowed. When other recording procedures are employed, adequate space must be provided for the length of the observation period.

Finally, regardless of the measurement procedure used, every data-recording form should include space for basic information such as the client's name and age, the therapist or observer's name, the date, the time, and the setting of the observation, and the behavior or performance event to be observed. Space should be left on the recording form to summarize the data in terms of totals or percentages.

Step 5: Record and Plot the Data Collected

Data obtained during the baseline period, during the treatment, and following the intervention are usually plotted on a graph or chart as a pictorial method for presenting the results. Line and bar graphs are the two most commonly used methods of plotting data. Both types of graphs have vertical and horizontal axes. The horizontal axis usually identifies the time period that the evaluation covers; it is typically divided into hours, days, or weeks. The vertical axis usually denotes the criteria used to evaluate treatment effects, i.e., increases or decreases in the performance of a defined behavior. Sufficient space should be allowed on both axes to accommodate the highest frequency of response and the longest period of time that may be required during the treatment. The space given to each measurement interval on both the horizontal and vertical axis should be large enough to visually convey the behavioral changes taking place during intervention. The visual interpretation and analysis of graphed data are discussed in Chapter 7.

Recording client performance may involve the construction of relatively simple line graphs or frequency charts, as described previously, or may involve the recording of the client's behavior on more detailed standardized charts which are commercially available. The Standard Behavior Chart is an example of a more detailed chart (Figure 4.1). It allows the therapist to chart recorded data in a very systematic, standardized manner (White and Haring, 1980).

Figure 4.1 is divided into semilog units, which is a format selected because of its utility in the estimation of linear trends in data and the ease with which it can be used by practitioners. Behaviors with extremely high or low rates can be recorded on the chart. The rates of behavior can vary from once in 24 hours to a maximum of 1,000 per minute. Behavior can be continuously recorded on the chart for up to 20 weeks. The wide range of rates that can be accepted by the chart enhances the accuracy of the recordings, since virtually no data are lost to ceiling or floor effects. Despite the apparent complexity of the chart it is a relatively simple and very accurate method of recording rates of behavior. White and Haring (1980) provide detailed instructions on the procedures involved in using the Standard Behavior Chart. In addition, Carr and Williams (1982) have provided some therapeutic examples of how the chart may be used to record data in a clinical setting.

Step 6: Continue Measurement and Recording Procedures until Requirements of the Design Have Been Satisfied

Once the measurement procedures have been developed, the final step is to continue observation and recording of client behavior until the desired change has occurred or until the requirements of the design have been satisfied. The design protocol for most single system investigations will include more than one phase. It is important that accurate measurements continue to be taken over the entire length of the evaluation period. The analysis and interpretation of the data collected can only be as good as the method of observation and recording that was used to collect the data. If the observation and recording procedures are vaguely defined or the data are carelessly recorded, any accurate interpretation of the effectiveness of the intervention will be impossible.

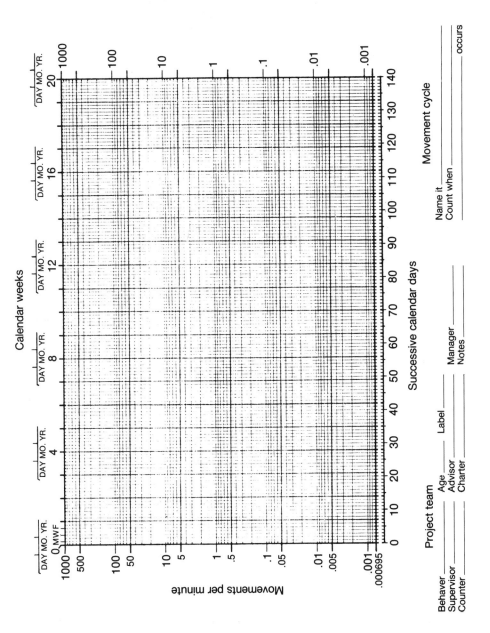

Figure 4.1. Example of the Standard Behavior Chart used to systematically record performance or behavior. (From: White, O. R., and Haring, N. G. (1980). *Exceptional Teaching* (2nd ed.). Columbus, OH, Charles E. Merrill.)

ISSUES IN MEASUREMENT AND
——————————— RECORDING ———————————

With use of single subject methods, therapists often have a choice among several options of the way data are to be collected. There are multiple dimensions along which therapists have choices among measurement and recording procedures. No procedure is always preferable. At best, the person responsible for the evaluation makes a conscious tradeoff; at worst, the therapist unwittingly biases the data.

Some evaluation and treatment questions require very precise, fine-grained, directly measured data, while other questions may be answered with data that are much less precise and indirect. It should not be assumed, however, that imprecise and fine-tuned data will provide the same degree of evidence or lead to the same conclusions. Manual muscle test results may not correspond closely to the results of more precise EMG testing. Usually, the more precise the data, the more expensive in both time and resources the data are to collect. The precision of assessment methods varies along a continuum from relatively imprecise to extremely precise. As an example, post hoc ratings, screening tests, diagnostic tests, and systematically gathered observations represent different points on a precision continuum.

Barlow et al. (1984) identify measures at one end of the continuum as molar. Molar measures include global or general ratings of behavior or performance. Many rating scales or screening instruments employed by therapists would be considered molar measures. At the other end of the continuum are molecular measures which represent the quantification of the occurrence or duration of specific behaviors. The amount or duration of direct eye contact exhibited by a depressed client in a group therapy session would be considered a molecular measure.

Regardless of whether the behaviors to be measured are classified as molar or molecular, there are a variety of ways that they may be measured. The emphasis in this chapter is on systematic direct observation of a client's performance by a therapist or other observer. This procedure is most commonly used when data on client performance is being collected in clinical settings. Other methods of data collecting are available, however. A common method of measurement in traditional group-comparison research is to employ standardized assessments, particularly norm-referenced standardized tests. Sometimes, standardized tests may be used as adjunct data collection devices in single system designs. The primary disadvantage of most standardized norm-referenced assessments is that they are difficult or impossible to administer on a repeated basis.

Bloom and Fischer (1982) advocate the use of self-anchored rating scales and client logs to collect data for some types of single system evaluation research. Self-anchored rating scales or client logs are particularly useful when the behavior to be measured is difficult to define in operational terms. With a self-anchored rating scale a continuum is devised on which the client rates his or her own behavior or performance. For example, suppose the purpose of a biofeedback and relaxation program is to reduce pain. A reduction in pain is difficult to operationally define, and a self-anchored rating scale may be developed to record the outcome of therapy. The client simply is asked to think of the worst pain he or she has ever experienced or can imagine and call this 100 pain units. The client then thinks of or imagines the state of absolute pain-free relaxation and calls this 0 pain units. This provides a scale ranging from 0 to 100 on which the client is taught to evaluate how much pain he or she is experiencing at any given moment.

Self-anchored scales or self-reports can be constructed for a variety of outcome measures and, depending on the nature of the client and the problem, are unique. Self-anchored rating scales may be used to operationally define problems and outcomes before and during intervention. It should be stressed, however, that self-anchored rating scales and other forms of self-report have a number of limitations. The first choice for a measurement or recording procedure should be influenced by consideration of what measure will give the "best" and most valuable information. The best information is that which is valid, reliable and useful. Because of their relatively greater effect on these three dimensions, any directly observable, measurable behaviors that are related to the client's actual functioning and that can be identified and systematically recorded should be considered first. If such directly observable behaviors do not exist, indirect measures such as self-anchored rating scales or other methods of self-reporting including client logs, on condition that their limitations are recognized and understood, can provide the therapist with valuable information.

Client self-report rating scales can be particularly useful in measuring the intensity of a disorder, as is suggested by the example of a self-anchored scale to report pain. Self-reports can also be used to evaluate internal thoughts and feelings or the intensity of those thoughts and feelings (Wolf, 1978). Thus, thoughts and feelings such as fears, excitement, depression, self-concept and other emotions can be evaluated. Smith and Kendall (1963) provide useful guidelines and suggestions for developing self-anchored rating scales with empirically formulated anchors.

The methodological issues related to the use of self-reports have seldom been addressed (Ysseldyke et al., 1973). The use of systematic direct observations, which are commonly employed in single system evaluation research, has been widely studied, however. Suggestions for the appropriate use of frequency counts, duration recording, or time sampling strategies have been offered in several introductory texts dealing with behavioral assessment (Cooper, 1981b; Hersen and Barlow, 1976; Kazdin, 1980).

Repp et al. (1976) have shown that the frequency and duration of responses may interact with various time sampling plans in such a way that the observation system distorts the data under various circumstances. Therapists may wish to consult one of the previously mentioned sources to obtain more information on such an interaction.

An important factor related to the general accuracy of measurement and recording is reactivity. Reactivity refers to "changes in the subject's sensitivity or responsiveness to treatment" (Campbell and Stanley, 1963) or to changes in the behavior due to the assessment process. Reactivity can affect the outcome of treatment, the actual implementation of the intervention, and the measurement or evaluation of each. The reactive effects of measurement can be temporary or permanent. Reactivity occurs when factors associated with the measurement process function as stimuli for change rather than as passive records of behavior (Haynes and Horn, 1982).

Assessment often affects the outcome of an intervention program. An evaluation designed to assess follow-up of activities taught to parents as part of an early intervention program may, for example, sensitize the parents to patterns of development. Parent knowledge may change as a result of the evaluation and may effect subsequent implementation of the intervention activities. On the other hand, play activities between handicapped and nonhandicapped school children may increase in the presence of an outside observer. In the first example, the reactive effects are permanent. In the second illustration, reactive effects may only be temporary.

The treatment itself may also be affected by the assessment process. Reactivity may affect measurement of the outcome for a particular treatment program. Some research indicates that when observers of a behavior are aware that their ability to accurately record behavior is being monitored (interobserver agreement), their assessment behavior changes; observers may apply definitional rules more strictly (Talpin and Reid, 1973) and be more conservative in recording target behaviors (Reid, 1970). The most obvious strategy for minimizing reactivity associated with interobserver agreement is to standardize the conditions under which assessment and agreement on assessment are conducted (Kazdin, 1979). Detailed suggestions for evaluating and dealing with the problem of reactivity are described by Kazdin (1982).

Undoubtedly, some inaccuracies in the measurement or evaluation of treatment outcomes can be attributed directly to recording errors. Therapists may accurately perceive and judge an event as having occurred, yet score or record that event as not having occurred. Several related factors may influence the probability of recording errors for both direct and indirect methods of measurement. These include measurement procedure, the complexity of the recording system, and the schedule for data collection.

In vivo recordings may involve therapists or other observers sampling behavior for brief periods (e.g., 30-second intervals) or extended durations (several hours). The opportunity to record observations can vary from several seconds to relatively unlimited time. For example, when videotapes are available and can be replayed as many times as needed, a relatively unlimited amount of time is available for accurate observations. In these cases, behaviors that are difficult to classify may be observed until they can be accurately scored. The therapist's time, for classifying and recording client performance, however, typically is limited. As a result, accuracy may be affected.

The complexity of a recording procedure also can influence accuracy. Observers may be required to record the presence or absence of discrete behaviors, to apply complex definitions of behaviors, to assess several responses simultaneously, or to record responses while maintaining a level of rapport with the client. Measurement complexity can be minimized by use of clearly formatted data sheets, behavior counters, electronic data recorders, and other equipment designed to simplify the task of recording complex behaviors. Incomplete and imprecise markings or recordings can be reduced with carefully designed coding systems and data-recording sheets. Behavior counters and electronic data recorders should be simple to use, and the observer should have experience with the apparatus prior to data collection.

Finally, schedules should be designed with some consideration of the factors that influence observer attention and concentration. These include the total time that any observer is expected to collect data in a given time period, the length of individual observation sessions, the nature of the observation task, and the experience and motivation of the therapist or persons serving as observers. Such factors can potentially influence the accuracy of recordings and thus threaten valid interpretations of the data collected.

ENSURING ACCURATE OBSERVATIONS AND MEASUREMENTS

A primary means of ensuring the accuracy of observations and measurements in single system evaluation and research is repeated measurements. As noted in the previous chapter, one of the fundamental principles of single systems strategies is repeated measurement of an individual's behavior over time, whether these behaviors be physiological reactions, motor movements, or psychological responses. In contrast to group comparison designs, in which only a few observations are taken (pretest-posttest), single system strategies require the frequent assessment of client behavior across time. Estimates based on these frequent measurements can be made concerning the degree of variability in a particular behavior of interest, its level of occurrence, and any apparent trends. These estimates are then used to determine the effectiveness or impact of treatment. The frequency of the observations and measurements obviously helps to ensure their accuracy.

It is impossible to know which clients improved in treatment and by how much unless frequent measures are taken of the individual receiving services. This point is often missed in discussions of the relative advantages of single system versus group-comparison designs. In the typical group-comparison design in which a premeasure and postmeasure are taken for subjects in both treatment and control groups, measurement error and other extraneous variables are totally inseparable from the treatment effect for any given individual. Thus, if client X improves 25 percent on a particular performance measure from pretest to posttest, it is impossible to determine if this improvement is due to variability in the measurement procedure, to maturational or other extraneous factors, or to the treatment itself.

Whether a therapist is doing single system evaluation or group-comparison research, the full determination of which specific individuals improved requires repeated assessment. In the clinical arena this is overtly understood. No experienced clinical therapist would be satisfied, over a period of time, with only one or two assessments of a client that included the determination of client needs and the design, implementation and conclusion of treatment. Suppose, for example, a physician took your blood pressure during an examination and found that it was above normal. If, relying on that one measurement, he then proceeded to develop a detailed plan of treatment, including drug therapy and possible hospitalization, you would probably feel that such measures were not justified based on a single recording of blood pressure. If the physician further informed you that no additional assessment of blood pressure would be taken until the treatment had been in effect for 2 weeks, you might seriously question his medical judgment. This same pretest-posttest method of determining clinical change is routinely applied in research designs in which group-comparison methods are used. For the practicing therapist dealing with the individual client, this type of decision-making approach is simply not acceptable.

Therapists are aware that the more frequently measures are taken, the higher the degree of precision (Barlow et al., 1984). If a therapist records behavior very infrequently, a determination of how much variability exists in the measure due to measurement error and extraneous variables may take a long time. The number of design options that the therapist can use to evaluate treatment will be limited, and the ability to discern treatment impact will be correspondingly restricted.

On the other hand, it is possible to record performance too frequently. This is particularly true when the measures are intrusive or are susceptible to factors such as practice or failure. Also, many measures are lengthy or difficult to administer and preclude frequent assessment. Usually, the solution for these problems is to take some measures frequently (those which are easy to implement, fairly unobtrusive, and likely to be agreed to by the client) and to supplement these with measures that can only be taken infrequently. If the measures are related, the more frequent measurement will tend to validate and support the less frequent measurement. For example, a therapist working with a client who has suffered a stroke may not be able to do a comprehensive assessment of motor skills frequently. These comprehensive evaluations may take several hours, and it is therefore not practical to repeat them too often. The therapist could, however, take a simple range of motion measure on an affected extremity which could then tend to validate the less frequently taken overall assessment and the less frequently taken overall assessment could tend to validate more frequently taken measure on the affected limb.

Reliability

As noted previously in this chapter, the observation and recording system used in single system evaluation research must be systematic. That is, particular measures of applied interest must be taken under similar conditions and must be recorded consistently. Any condition that might reasonably be expected to influence the measurement cannot be allowed to vary with the treatment. Usually, the best way to protect against this is to keep the measurement and observation procedure as standard as possible on such dimensions as the time of assessment, the observer, implicit demands on the client, and the like. An issue closely related to systematic measurement of client performance is the reliability of the measurement procedures. In many single system designs, measurement relies on the observation of a specific target behavior. It makes little sense to develop a sophisticated systematic method of coding performance, such as the Standard Behavior Chart described previously, if the therapist or individual doing the recording is poorly trained or unreliable in his or her recording activities. The behavior to be recorded must be clearly defined, and the recorder or observer must be familiar with how, when, where, and how long the behavior should be observed and recorded.

In clinical environments the observation and recording of a client's performance is often accomplished by the therapist, an aide, or whoever can be conveniently recruited to participate in the activity. Tawney and Gast (1984) suggest that the following guidelines be followed when one is training or recruiting persons to function as observers and recorders of client behavior. Ideally, the observer should not be aware of the purpose of the investigation, nor should he or she know the status of the client in relation to the design, i.e., whether the client is in the baseline phase or in the intervention phase. Second, the observer should have had some training and instruction prior to observing and recording the patient's behavior. Ideally, the observer has had the opportunity to practice recording the behavior prior to the initiation of the evaluation. Also, the conditions under which training and practice occurred should be a close approximation to those of the actual treatment or recording environment. If more than one observer or recorder is to be employed, the amount of communication between them should be minimal to eliminate possible bias or confusion regarding the performance being measured. Finally, the reliability of the observers and recording system should be checked during the course of the investigation to determine the accuracy and consistency of the measurement and recording plan.

Numerous methods are available to evaluate the reliability of observers. Percentage agreement procedures are widely recommended for calculating interobserver reliability in applied or clinical settings (Bijou et al., 1968; Hawkins and Dotson, 1975). Percentage agreement scores can be calculated for the total number of observations during a session, regardless of the method of data collection employed in a given evaluation. This method is most frequently employed with frequency, duration or rate measures (Kelly, 1977). Estimates of total reliability are obtained by simply dividing the smaller score recorded by one observer with the larger score recorded by a second observer. The resultant ratio is then multiplied by 100, and a percentage of agreement is obtained. For example, if two observers recorded the time that a child with cerebral palsy was able to maintain an upright sitting posture, one observer might record 45 seconds of correct sitting over a 5-minute period, while a second observer might record 50 seconds of correct sitting over the same time period. Obviously, the criteria for ''correct sitting'' would have been previously defined and agreed on by both observers. With use of the procedure described above,

$$\frac{45}{50} = .90 \times 100 = 90\%.$$

An interrater agreement of 90% would have been found for the response of correct sitting.

The total percentage method of calculating interobserver reliability is easy to compute and has intuitive appeal but has a number of limitations, and several authorities have recommended that it not be used to compute interobserver agreement (Jackson and Wallace, 1974; Johnson and Bolstad, 1973). The argument has been made that reliability methods based on total number of responses are inadequate because they do not provide information regarding agreement on individual occurrences of behavior. Two observers could obtain perfect agreement on the total number or duration of the responses produced, despite having recorded entirely different occurrences of the behavior.

Suppose, for instance, that in the previous example the first observer recorded the 45 seconds of correct sitting behavior in the first 2 minutes of the 5-minute trial period, while the second observer recorded 50 seconds of correct sitting behavior in the last 3 minutes of the 5-minute trial period. Obviously, the observers were not in agreement. That is, they were not reliably recording the same target behavior, yet the percentage agreement based on total responses is at a very acceptable level (90%). The 90% agreement between the two observers indicates that the observers agree on the total duration (or frequency) of the behavior with a 10% (100% minus 90%) margin of error. It does not mean that the observers agree 90% of the time. Although one observer recorded 45 seconds of correct sitting and the other recorded 50 seconds, there is no way of knowing whether they recorded the same responses (Harris and Lahey, 1978).

In an attempt to circumvent the inadequacies of "total" response reliability procedures, many clinicians obtain observer agreement on the occurrence and nonoccurrence of target behaviors on a response-by-response basis. This is perhaps the most widely used method of calculating observer agreement in the single system or within-subject research literature (Kelly, 1977). This method, sometimes referred to as point-to-point reliability, provides an indication of the consistency and accuracy of recording for individual responses and, therefore, is closely related to the basic premise of single system evaluation and research (Bloom and Fischer, 1982). In addition, the formula used for determining the percentage of agreement is easy to apply. Unlike correlational or other frequently advocated procedures, this method does not require a semisophisticated understanding of statistics.

For calculation of this form of interobserver agreement, two observers independently record the behavior of a client according to a predetermined response definition of what constitutes appropriate performance. After the period of observation, the records are examined on a response-by-response basis to determine the number of agreements and disagreements present for both occurrences and nonoccurrences (or errors) of the target behavior. When this approach is used, an agreement is defined as concurrence between observers that a response did or did not occur on a given trial or during a given recording interval. Alternately, disagreements reflect instances in which one observer recorded an occurrence of an acceptable response, while a second did not.

In the earlier example in which correct sitting was the target behavior, the 5-minute trial period might be broken down into ten recording intervals of 30 seconds each. During each of the intervals the observers are required to place a plus (+) on the recording form if correct sitting occurred or to place a minus $(-)$ if the target behavior did not occur during that 30-second interval. Table 4.1 displays the possible outcome on a response-by-response basis. The intervals (trials) for which disagreement occurred are indicated by an asterisk (*). It can be seen from the Table 4.1 that there are a total of 8 agreements and 2 disagreements for the ten 30-second intervals. The following formula is used to compute the percentage of interobserver agreement:

$$\frac{\text{Total number of agreements}}{\text{Total number of agreements plus disagreements}}$$
$$\times\ 100\ =\ \text{Percentage of agreement.}$$

If the data from Table 4.1 are inserted into the formula,

$$\frac{8}{(8\ +\ 2)} = .80 \times 100 = 80\%,$$

an interobserver agreement of 80% would be obtained.

The response-by-response method of interobserver agreement has considerable practical utility. It also has some limitations, however. The basic weakness of this method is that the agreement level obtained is a direct reflection of the rate of production of the target behavior. That is, when the response-by-response method is used and the rate of the target behavior is either very high or very low, observers are fairly certain to reach high levels of interobserver agreement (Bijou et al., 1968). Despite this limitation the response-by-response method of measuring interobserver agreement remains a very useful tool for establishing the reliability of recording and measurement procedures in single system evaluation.

Obviously, reliability is a crucial issue in single system evaluation research, as it is in all research. Consistent observation and recording of

Table 4.1.
Data Depicting Interobserver Agreement for Two Observers

30-second interval	Observer 1	Observer 2	Disagreements
1	+	+	
2	−	+	*
3	+	+	
4	+	+	
5	+	+	
6	+	−	*
7	−	−	
8	−	−	
9	+	+	
10	+	+	

client performance are crucial for accurate assessment. Without reliable assessment it will be difficult or impossible to know just what the client's actual performance was. If measurements and recordings are not reliable, any change in performance may be a reflection of some modification or fluctuation in the recording of the behavior, rather than a result of an actual change in the client's behavior. Finally, high reliability ensures that the behavior is clearly and well defined. Thus, the intervention can be more efficiently and effectively implemented.

There are multiple reasons for poor reliability in measuring or recording behavior (Martin and Pear, 1978). The definition of the target behavior might be vague or incomplete. The behavior might be difficult to observe because of problems or distractions in the observational environment or because the behavior to be recorded is subtle and hard to detect. The observer might be poorly trained or unmotivated. At the other extreme, the observer might be biased or might expect certain behaviors from the clients because of a vested interest in the treatment outcome or because of an assumption about how the client should behave. The reliability might be affected by use of instruments which are clumsy or poorly designed and difficult to use. Finally, there may be systematic changes in the way an observer records over time (observer drift) due to fatigue, disinterest, practice or some other factor. All of these and other variables may affect the reliability of the assessment of client performance. It is crucial to eliminate or control these events as much as possible and to evaluate the reliability of the observation and recording procedures being used in the evaluation of a treatment program.

CONCLUSION

Although this chapter is certainly not exhaustive of the subject, it provides descriptions of several prominent measurement and recording concerns that need to be addressed in any evaluation employing single system procedures. A review of evaluation and efficacy reports in occupational and physical therapy indicates the difficulty that therapists encounter in attempting to deal with these considerations. Major obstacles to adequate recording and measurement are limited resources, technical complications, unfamiliarity with the procedures and methodology, and lack of good models.

Therapists interested in evaluating their treatment programs must establish priorities and address those concerns which pose the greatest threats to accuracy, generalization, and interpretation of data. In the hierarchy of these threats, accuracy of recording and measurement seems a logical place to start. The preceding sections of this chapter have provided therapists with the basic information that they need to begin to accurately collect and record data related to therapeutic effectiveness.

The complexity of the assessment and evaluation process requires a flexibility of measurement and recording methods that is consistent with a wide variety of possible treatment outcomes. To achieve this end, therapists must regard measurement and recording not as nuisances or obstacles but as an integral part of the single system evaluation process.

CHAPTER 5

Basic Designs for Single System Evaluation and Research

————————————— **INTRODUCTION** —————————————

Clinical practice conducted within the framework of single system evaluation strategies can enhance the quality of therapeutic intervention. The designs associated with single system methods involve a set of procedural guidelines for the empirical measurement of clinical intervention with a single client or small group of patients. The assessment of client function occurs over a period of time and provides repeated measures of at least one problem or goal throughout the treatment process. Although overt behaviors are generally the object of study, any feeling or experience which can be defined and provided with a behavioral or empirical referent can be measured and evaluated with use of single system procedures. The designs presented in this chapter provide the basic framework for collecting data in a systematic and reliable fashion compatible with the clinically based use of single system evaluation procedures.

The single system methodology provides a flexible framework for the incorporation of scientific methods into the clinical practice setting. As such, the process and logic associated with single system designs closely parallels that found in traditional "experimental" investigations. In the single system design, reliable and valid data are collected repeatedly over a period of time. Data collected when the intervention is in effect are compared with data collected when the intervention is not in effect. These no-treatment periods or baselines allow the client to function as his or her own control or standard of comparison. Via this general framework, single system methodology contributes to at least two major goals: (1) monitoring of client progress and (2) determination of whether the treatment was responsible for improved performance.

The single system model is not a fixed procedure but is a collection of procedures or guidelines that may be used to serve several purposes. One of the goals that a therapist might have could be to demonstrate a degree of "experimental control" for a particular intervention over a given target behavior. That is, the clinician may wish to establish a cause-effect relationship between two or more variables. For other therapists, demonstration of this relationship may not be a high priority. The majority of clinicians may be more interested in simply monitoring a client's progress over time. Whatever the clinician's priorities in a particular case, the knowledge of single system evaluation strategies adds important potential benefits to a therapist's practice repertoire. The application of single system methods allows the therapist to make a useful contribution, with each client, to a professional and/or personal body of knowledge regarding the effects of clinical interventions.

The initial advantage of single system designs in clinical practice is derived simply from the process of defining relevant problems and goals in clearly specified and measurable terms. This process provides a framework for both the client and therapist to consider the need for intervention, the intended goals of treatment, and any possible desirable or undesirable side effects. Although different types of problems and goals will be specified in different ways, depending on the client's specific needs and the therapist's practice style, the overall method associated with the systematic development of a single system design can help clarify the treatment process for all concerned.

Therapeutic effectiveness should be enhanced because repeated empirical feedback associated with single system designs allows the therapist and client to accurately monitor the ongoing progress, or lack of progress, and to respond appropriately. Continuous feedback regarding the client's behavior or performance prior to intervention (baseline) can provide useful information about the extent of the problem. For example, it may be determined during the baseline period that the originally identified problem is not as severe as first described, and intervention targeted at another problem area may be more appropriate.

Feedback after intervention has been in effect for a period of time can provide information that the therapist can use to make judgments about continuing, discontinuing or, in some way, altering the intervention. In addition, ongoing feedback to the client regarding his or her progress can be a key ingredient leading to a desirable outcome. Providing clients with a graphic record or demonstration of progress can encourage continuation of treatment when perceived change is slow. It may also help the client discriminate those instances when positive change has occurred and may lead to information on which successful replications can be based.

Obviously, for the client and therapist to obtain the maximum benefit from the use of single system methodology, the specific design to be employed and its strengths and weaknesses must be clearly understood. Single system designs may be viewed on a continuum of control. At one end of the continuum are those design strategies which provide relatively little in the way of systematically planned comparisons across conditions or phases. These "designs," often referred to as case studies, rely primarily on observation and systematic description. At the other end of the single system design continuum are a number of very complex designs emphasizing planned and controlled comparisons of client performance across various phases, settings, or individuals. These designs are considered very "powerful," since causal inferences based on the results can be drawn. The remainder of this chapter and Chapter 6 are devoted to explaining and illustrating some designs associated with the single system continuum.

CASE STUDY DESIGNS

Practicing therapists are intuitively aware that generally the accumulation of evidence about the effects of a given intervention is accomplished gradually. Early research efforts are often exploratory in nature and rely on the in-depth or intense description of the individual case, while later efforts are often designed in accordance with what is found in these early empirical activities.

In their classic text on research designs, Campbell and Stanley (1963) outline the premise that designs lie on a continuum ranging from designs that are exploratory in nature and offer tentative data concerning an intervention, to intensive highly controlled "true" experiments that permit the researcher to draw inferences about the causal effects of interventions. Acceptance of a continuum of research methods and investigative procedures designed both to elaborate and explore phenomena at one end of the continuum and to provide convincing demonstration of causal relationships at the other end helps to reconcile the objectives of research and clinical practice. Cook and Campbell (1979, p. 15) have pointed out that there are many possible conceptions of causality and that "observed causal relationships in the social sciences will be fallible rather than inevitable and that the connections between antecedents and consequences will be probabilistic."

If the goals of single system evaluation and research are broadly conceived as the exploration of probabilistic causal connections and the objective monitoring of client performance, their ultimate achievement should not be threatened by the use of a wide range of single system strategies including exploratory case studies. A case study generally includes an in-depth investigation and a description of an individual or small group. In a typical case study, information is collected from a multitude of sources over a period of time. In the rehabilitation fields, case studies are typically conducted to determine the background, environment and characteristics of individuals with a handicapping condition. The primary purpose of a case study is to determine the factors, and the relationships among a set of variables, which have resulted in the current disability or status of the person under study. In other words, the purpose of most case studies is to determine what a person's status is. The case study methodology does not allow the therapist to establish functional relationships between the various factors being described.

In its simplest form the case study consists of systematically recorded observations of an individual patient. The case study usually includes information derived from the assessment or treatment of a particular client. The information is reported in much detail, so that the narrative description captures as much as possible of the unique characteristics of the individual client and his or her treatment, behavior or setting. In occupational and physical therapy the case study is typically conducted in the context of treatment. The case study provides an elaborate description of the individual. Inferences based on this description may be drawn about factors in the client's past, present or future that are likely to account for current performance. The information from which these inferences are derived is usually anecdotal and includes clinical impressions, judgments, and assumptions made by the therapist.

Cox and West (1982, p. 26) observe that the "case study is a descriptive research design, the primary purpose of which is to describe in detail certain characteristics of the subject." They go on to note that although some case studies may contain "experimental aspects," these studies typically do not include planned comparisons between conditions or phases or attempt to control or manipulate treatment or outcome measures. As a result, there is seldom any concern with issues related to measurement or the recording of predetermined client behaviors. Nevertheless, the case study method can provide the therapist with valuable information related to client performance. Cubie and Kaplan (1982) argue that a well-described and -developed case study, particularly if it is associated with an identifiable frame of reference, can provide the practicing clinician with a valuable problem-solving strategy for treating individual clients. A well-developed case study can provide information and a rationale for the use of a particular treatment technique and can result in the generation of client case records that may be useful for future clinical research and the documentation of services.

Kazdin (1980) has identified four functions of the well-constructed case study in a clinical environment. These functions include (1) a source of ideas and hypotheses about patient performance, (2) a source of information regarding specific or unique applications of therapeutic procedures, (3) the ability to study a rare phenomenon, and (4) the ability to provide a counterinstance of a generally accepted proposition or finding.

The first function cited by Kazdin (1980) is to provide ideas and hypotheses for further study. This is a frequently identified function of the case study. In this capacity, the case study is viewed as a method for investigating an area that has not been subjected to previous empirical inquiry. A hypothesis based on the results of a thorough description of an individual case can then be subjected to study with use of a procedure that will allow the investigator more confidence in the conclusions than can be achieved through the uncontrolled case study.

In the second application described by Kazdin (1980), the case study may suggest how a particular therapeutic strategy may be modified for use in a new or unique situation. The extension of a specific therapy procedure to a new problem is a common occurrence in clinical practice and may be facilitated by conducting a well-designed case study. For example, a therapist might present a case study describing the application of transcutaneous nerve stimulation (TENS) to reduce the incidence of stereotypic or self-injurious behavior in a patient with severe developmental disability. A successful case study describing the application of TENS, administered as a form of sensory stimulation designed to reduce self-injurious behavior, would clearly represent the extension of an established therapeutic procedure to a new problem area.

The case study method also provides the framework for studying a rare phenomenon or clinical case, which is the third function identified by Kazdin (1980). Many of the disabilities encountered in clinical environments are unusual and will never occur in large enough numbers to be systematically studied with use of traditional group-comparison methods. The case study provides a procedure for gathering information about low-incidence clinical phenomena. The rare clinical case can be intensively studied with use of the case study method, and information may be obtained that will lead to a better understanding of the phenomenon or a more efficient treatment approach.

The fourth and final function of a case study as described by Kazdin (1980) is to provide a counterinstance of a commonly held proposition that is believed to be universally applicable. As a technique for disproving a generally accepted finding, the case study may be very useful. For example, suppose there was a syndrome that was widely considered to be sex-linked recessive in nature and manifest only in males. A case study carefully documenting the signs and symptoms of the disorder in a female patient would cast doubt on the general belief that the syndrome occurs only in males. By demonstration of counterinstance, the case study can provide a qualifier regarding the generality of a proposition or commonly held belief.

Case studies frequently appear in the rehabilitation literature. Individual studies labeled as case reports appear as a regular feature in *Physical Therapy*. Lucci (1980) has published a compilation of 41 clinical cases entitled, *Occupational Therapy Case Studies*. These sources provide valuable descriptive information concerning the clients served by therapists and also provide data related to documentation. Because planned comparisons are not made across different conditions or phases and the intervention is not systematically manipulated, however, descriptive case studies do not provide the "best" source for objectively documenting clinical change or for providing evidence of treatment effectiveness.

Connolly et al. (1983) differentiate between three types of single-case approaches to answering clinical questions. The three forms are (1) the single-case description, also called the single-case report; (2) the single-case study; and (3) the single-case design investigation. The single-case design investigation involves the manipulation of a treatment and the systematic recording of client performance over planned phases. This description corresponds to many of the single system designs discussed in later sections of this chapter and throughout the remainder of the text. The differentiation between the single-case description or report and the single-case study is the topic of immediate concern. Connolly et al. (1983, p. 1767) define the single-case description as "a detailed documentation and summary of the characteristics, diagnosis, problem, treatment, and response of one patient." This description may include a detailed narrative of the client's inpatient and outpatient history and status, including observation, and measurements taken before, during and after treatment. Because no planned comparisons or manipulations of the intervention are conducted and no systematic attempt is made to define and record patient performance within a design structure, however, the results of the single-case description cannot be used to support or demonstrate the effectiveness of an intervention.

The single-case study as defined by Connolly et al. (1983) includes the same type of descriptive information as the single-case description; in addition, the single-case study contains a review of the literature. In the single-case study as described by Connolly et al. (1983), a detailed narrative account of the patient's history, current status and performance is integrated with the relevant literature, and appropriate comparisons and contrasts can then be made between the case presented and other related case studies.

Because of the limitations referred to earlier, the simple descriptive case study should not be expected to provide accurate and reliable information about the effectiveness of a particular intervention. Nor is the case study the ideal method to use for monitoring client progress. A more systematic approach, which is associated with the designs presented throughout the rest of this chapter and in Chapter 6, is required to achieve these objectives.

AB DESIGNS

The most basic single system strategy that employs a planned comparison is referred to as the AB design. The AB design consists of initially establishing a pattern of client responses for a specific target behavior, then implementing a change in conditions, usually the introduction of the treatment, while maintaining the measurement procedures. The client's response patterns are then reviewed and analyzed for both the pre-intervention and intervention phases. This is referred to as the within-series or within-subject strategy, since systematic changes obtained within a series of data points across time for a single client are examined.

The "A" in the AB design represents the baseline or the no-treatment condition, while the "B" refers to the first identified treatment or intervention phase. Subsequent interventions are indicated by different letters of the alphabet. If an intervention or baseline is repeated, the same letter is used to represent the repeated phase.

In the typical AB design, the therapist uses the first phase or baseline to help determine or illustrate the phenomenon of interest and to develop a standard of performance. Against this background the therapist can then examine the client's response pattern demonstrated in the second phase when the intervention is introduced. If there are major changes in the expected pattern of performance from the baseline through the first intervention phase, the therapist may logically suspect that an effect has occurred.

For example, Figure 5.1 displays the effect of an oral motor intervention program on the weight gain of a profoundly mentally retarded student. In this study, it was hypothesized that an increase or improvement in oral-motor function and feeding ability in severely handicapped persons would result in an increase in weight gain (Ottenbacher et al., 1983). The student whose response patterns are depicted in Figure 5.1 was a 10-year 11-month-old boy diagnosed as profoundly mentally retarded. The student was a

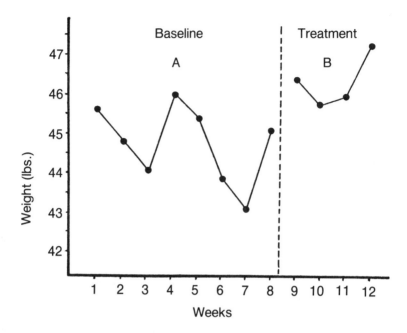

Figure 5.1. Example of AB design showing baseline and treatment phases. The graph illustrates changes in weight over the baseline period (A) and the period of oral motor intervention (B) for a mentally retarded student.

resident of a state-supported hospital and was identified as a problem feeder by the residential staff. He weighed only 45.6 pounds at the beginning of the study. The A phase of the design represents the baseline period in which the client's weight was recorded. The resident's weight was obtained twice weekly by an aide who was unaware of whether the student was in the baseline or intervention phase. The twice weekly recordings of weight were averaged and appear in the A phase of Figure 5.1. A program of oral-motor therapy, which is described in detail by Ottenbacher et al. (1983) and was designed to normalize muscle tone and reduce abnormal reflex activity, was initiated at the end of the eighth week of baseline and represents the B condition or intervention phase. The client's weight continued to be recorded in the same manner as described previously. The response patterns in Figure 5.1 for the two phases suggests that the resident's weight increased during the B phase of intervention.

In retrospect, the dependent or outcome measure used in this study may have not been sufficiently sensitive to reflect changes in oral-motor function and feeding ability. The measure of weight gain was selected because it could be blindly recorded and was felt to be an objective and reliable measure. Although these are definite advantages, it could be argued that the measure provided only an indirect indication of improvement in oral-motor function. Ray et al. (1983) conducted a related study in which a more "sensitive" and direct measure of oromotor function was employed. This study is described in more detail in the next section.

The selection of the most appropriate outcome measure often generates controversy and concern in applied research (Nelson, 1981). The earlier example is a good illustration of this point. The outcome measure of weight in pounds could be reliably and objectively recorded by a person unaware of the treatment procedures or the status of the client in relation to treatment. This is an obvious advantage; the possibility exists, however, that the measure was not directly sensitive to changes in oral-motor behavior. It is often very difficult to develop or identify an individualized outcome measure that can be accurately and reliably recorded and is still sensitive to changes in client performance. Therapists should strive to select outcome measures that meet both of these requirements. Sacrifices in either area will reduce the clinical usefulness of single system evaluation strategies.

The simple AB design described earlier can accomplish several goals. First, the AB design provides a framework for therapeutic accountability. This is important for a number of obvious reasons alluded to in previous chapters. The cornerstone of accountability is being able to give an accurate report of what the therapist did in treatment and what progress the client made. The AB design provides the mechanism to achieve this goal. As Bloom and Fischer (1982, p. 385) observe, "the fundamental step in becoming an accountable professional is to start counting with the AB design." The AB design provides a specific design framework for manipulating the treatment and outcome variable and requires that the treatment and outcome variable be clearly identified and operationally defined. As part of the operationalization of the dependent variable, the issue of measurement reliability must be addressed and a systematic method of observing and recording client performance must be developed.

The basic AB design also provides the foundation for tentative statements concerning the likelihood that improvement is directly due to treatment. Suppose, for example, that an AB design appears to show a clear treatment effect and that we know this same effect has been demonstrated on several other clients in a variety of clinical settings. In such a case, we may be fairly confident that the treatment effect with a particular client is real and not an artifact of the client or setting.

Our confidence in the results from an AB design is also increased if we know, based on other information, that a particular behavior is very resistant to change and not likely to be spontaneously modified. If, in addition, we have a long and stable baseline of preintervention responses, any dramatic effect following treatment implementation may be more confidently attributed to the intervention.

In most isolated cases in which the AB design is used, a change from A to B will need to be repeated either within the same client or across clients before the therapist can be sure of any treatment effect. The simple AB design does not control for a number of possible extraneous variables that might have produced an improvement or change in responses. As Tawney and Gast (1984) note, the most significant limitation of the isolated AB design is the lack of information on the natural course of ''change'' for the behavior of interest. Without such information, it is impossible to rule out the influence of uncontrolled variables (historical confounds) or the effects of the passage of time (maturation) on the target behavior.

The results of an AB design can be confirmed by replication. The generalization and strength of single system methods are based on replication as the ultimate source of confidence in the results obtained. The effect of an AB design can be replicated in many different ways, and the importance of replication is discussed in a later chapter. One common method of replication used with the simple AB design is to replicate one of the phases. In other words, the within-design replication would involve repeating one or more of the phases already introduced. This strategy would result in an ABA design or an ABAB design.

———— VARIATIONS OF THE AB DESIGN ————

ABA Design

The ABA design is simply a logical extension of the AB design in which the treatment is withdrawn in the third phase. The withdrawal of the intervention (the second A phase) provides greater confidence in the ability to determine the effect of the treatment based on what Barlow and Hersen (1973, p. 320) label ''the principle of unlikely successive coincidences.'' In other words, it is possible that a response pattern could change due to something other than the intervention, which could be coincidentally affecting the client's behavior or performance at approximately the same time that the treatment is introduced. With each successive pattern change corresponding to the introduction or withdrawal of the intervention, it becomes increasingly unlikely that any change in performance can be attributed to such a coincidence. As rival threats such as history and maturation are controlled for by the use of the withdrawal strategy introduced in the AB design, the strength of the design in terms of establishing a functional relationship between the treatment and client performance is improved. If other events external or internal to the client and not associated with the treatment were, in fact, responsible for any change in performance across the first two phases, the behavior would not be expected to revert to baseline levels during the second A phase.

Ray et al. (1983) used an ABA design to evaluate the effectiveness of techniques designed to facilitate mouth closure and, thus, decrease drooling in an 11-year-old boy identified as mentally retarded and with cerebral palsy. During the first baseline period, which lasted 2 weeks, the student engaged in 10 half-hour play sessions. Each play session was followed by a 1-hour period during which the client wore an absorbent bib. The amount of drooling was quantified by weighing the bib at the beginning of the hour and again at the end. The recorded outcome measure was the amount (weight) of saliva that was collected on the bib during the 1-hour period. During the intervention phase (B), which lasted 4 weeks, the half-hour play period was replaced by a half-hour period of treatment in which the client received specific oromotor therapy designed to improve mouth closure. Following the half hour of therapy, the amount of drooling was recorded over a 1-hour period in the same manner as during the baseline. The final phase (second A phase) consisted of a withdrawal of the oromotor therapy and a return to a half-hour play period identical to that used in the first baseline period. The amount of drooling continued to be recorded in the same manner as during the first baseline and intervention. The graphic results are presented in Figure 5.2 and clearly indicate that drooling diminished during the intervention phase. Ray et al. (1983, p. 749) concluded that the "results indicate that the amount of saliva leaving the mouth was a function of the presence or absence of intervention." The authors were careful to note, however, that their results were based on the performance of only one subject and cannot be generalized without additional replications. The study by Ray et al. (1983) provides an excellent example of the use of a single system strategy, the ABA design, to document the effectiveness of a therapeutic intervention procedure in a clinical setting.

Laskas et al. (1985) recently presented a clinically based ABA design. They examined the immediate effect of four neurodevelopmental treatment activities on the lower extremity functions of a young child with spastic quadriplegia. An EMG was used to measure dorsiflexor motor activity in the lower extremity across the three phases (ABA) of the design. Data on the frequency of heel contact during movement to a standing position were also collected over a number of trials. When these data were compared with data gathered in the baseline and nontreatment periods, an increase in dorsiflexor muscle activity and in heel contact during the treatment periods was demonstrated.

A potential limitation of the ABA design, which is evident in both of the examples presented previously, is that the ABA design begins with a baseline phase and leaves the client in an undesirable state, i.e., the absence of treatment. In some settings, this may be a major limitation to implementing such a design in a clinical setting (Thomas, 1979).

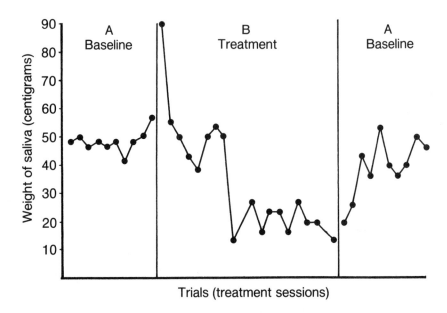

Figure 5.2. Line graph illustrating response pattern for ABA design. (Adapted from: Ray, S. A., Bundy, A. C., and Nelson, D. L. (1983). Decreasing drooling through techniques to facilitate mouth closure. *Am. J. Occup. Ther., 37,* 749–753.)

ABAB Design

A simple solution to this problem with the ABA design is to reintroduce the treatment and create an ABAB design. Procedurally, the design consists of a basic ABA approach extended by the addition of a final treatment phase. This modification is important because it overcomes a major ethical and practical limitation of the ABA design by ending with a treatment period rather than with a no-treatment phase. The ABAB design is likely to be more acceptable to therapists, clients, and administrators because it allows the evaluation to end with the client in an improved state. In addition, the ABAB design provides strong evidence of intervention effects, since the client's response to treatment is observed on two separate occasions. That is, if changes in the rate of client performance cooccur with application and reapplication of the intervention, it is highly probable that the change in client performance was functionally related to treatment.

Figure 5.3 presents a hypothetical data series for an ABAB design. The similarities between this design and the previously present AB and ABA designs should be obvious. Inspection of Figure 5.3 reveals that improvement in client performance occurred at the beginning of the initial treatment (B) phase and continued throughout this phase. The subsequent withdrawal

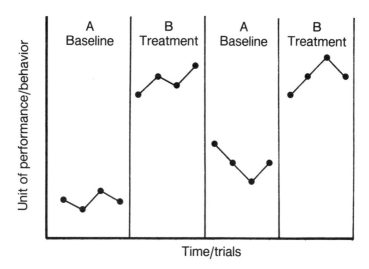

Figure 5.3. Example of an ABAB design illustrating response patterns across baseline and intervention phases. Data series shows an increase in performance during treatment periods and a corresponding decrease in performance during baseline phases.

of intervention is marked by a slight decline or reversal in client performance (second A phase). To this point, the design is essentially an ABA design, and sufficient evidence has been accumulated to suggest that the intervention is producing the desired therapeutic effect. Reinstatement of the treatment during the final phase of the evaluation (second B phase) and the associated increase in the client's response pattern, however, provides additional evidence that the increase in client performance was a result of the manipulation of the treatment. The correspondence between the manipulation of a treatment and the resultant change in client performance across the various phases in the ABAB design provides convincing evidence that treatment was effective in producing an improvement in the target behavior.

Sobsey and Orelove (1984) used an ABAB design to examine the effects of neurophysiological facilitation procedures on eating skills in four severely handicapped children. An ABAB design was employed to evaluate the effects of neurophysiologically based intervention on lip closure, rotary chewing, and the spilling of food and drink from the mouth. Some improvements were revealed in each of the four students when the facilitation procedures were administered. Figure 5.4 presents the percent of bites with lip closure across each of the four design phases for one of the subjects in this study. The response pattern for this particular child indicates that the introduction of the facilitation procedures during the two treatment phases

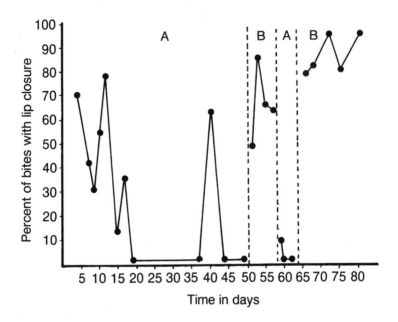

Figure 5.4. Percent of bites with lip closure during periods of intervention (B) and nonintervention (A). (Adapted from: Sosbey, R., and Orelove, F. P. (1984). Neurophysiological facilitation of eating skills in children with severe handicaps. *J. Assoc. Severely Handicapped, 9,* 102.)

(B), compared with the nonintervention phases, was associated with an improvement in lip closure.

A disadvantage of the ABA or the ABAB design is that if the intervention is successful and a change in behavior or performance occurs, it may not be possible to return to baseline during the second A phase. In other words, the behavior change associated with the intervention may be permanent. For example, if intervention designed to improve the range of motion (ROM) of a client with an elbow contracture is successful, it is not reasonable to expect that if the treatment is withdrawn, the client will immediately lose the range of motion gained and revert back to a contracted state. If a return to baseline performance when the intervention is withdrawn is impossible or unlikely, alternate design strategies, such as the multiple baseline strategy discussed in Chapter 6, may be more appropriate.

That a behavior does not return to baseline levels on withdrawal of the intervention does not, however, mean that the results based on an ABA or ABAB design have been compromised. If the behavior continues to improve during the second A phase, there will be little need to intervene further, since the client is obviously improving. The therapist may continue to record performance and the design becomes an AB design with the second A phase constituting a follow-up period. If no change is observed in the second A phase; i.e., the client's performance neither deteriorates nor continues to improve, several options are open to the therapist. Reinstating the treatment, i.e., extending the design to an ABAB, seems to be the most logical course of action in this case.

The complete reversal to baseline in an ABA or ABAB design is not a logical requirement of the design per se. The therapist employing single system strategies is typically interested in client improvement rather than in the achievement of some specified steady state of behavioral performance. The therapist is interested in demonstrating that intervention results in more client improvements than does nonintervention. Figure 5.5 presents data from an ABAB design in which the second A phase resulted in a leveling off of performance or a period of no change. As is clearly shown in Figure 5.5, when the treatment is reintroduced (second B phase), there is a continued improvement in client performance. Hayes (1981) presents a method of plotting data which is associated with a response pattern similar to that portrayed in Figure 5.5. The method allows the computation of a difference score based on trends established in the previous phase. When the data are plotted by use of this method, they show a classic "reversal" pattern in improvement, which is related to a trend rather than to an absolute level. The procedure proposed by Hayes (1981) is discussed in more detail in Chapter 7 which deals with the visual analysis of single system data. *Failure to return to baseline levels of performance in an ABA or an ABAB design, however, does not necessarily reduce the effectiveness of the design in monitoring client progress or in demonstrating the effectiveness of the intervention.*

BAB Design

Often, it is particularly difficult to delay introducing intervention in clinical environments while the baseline data are collected during the first A phase. Another variation of the AB design and an alternative to the previously discussed ABA or ABAB designs is the BAB design. This design may be particularly useful in those instances in which it is not possible to initially collect baseline data. After the intervention has been introduced, a "baseline" phase (without treatment) may be justified to determine whether the intervention effects will be maintained. Figure 5.6 displays the response pattern from a BAB design. In this case, the outcome measure was defined as the client's ability to sip and swallow liquid from a cup without any loss. The client's performance was recorded in terms of percent correct responses per day and then was averaged for each week of the evaluation. The first phase (B) represents an intervention condition in

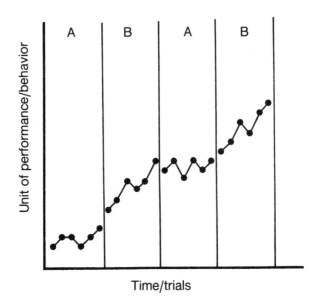

Figure 5.5.   Line graph illustrating ABAB design with a leveling off of the response pattern during the second A phase.

which jaw control techniques and positioning of the head were initiated during the drinking of liquids. The response pattern in this phase represents the client's performance during intervention. In the second phase (A), jaw control procedures and positioning of the head were withdrawn. Responses during the second phase reveal the client's response pattern associated with a period of no intervention. The responses in the A phase represent a delayed ''baseline'' which can be used to compare performance during the intervention periods. Finally, in the third phase the treatment (jaw control and positioning) was reintroduced. The response pattern in Figure 5.6 clearly demonstrates a change in the client's performance across the phases.

The major advantages of the BAB design are its ability to evaluate ongoing treatment and its lack of requirement of an initial baseline. The A phase or withdrawal of treatment in the BAB design may occur as a natural function of the treatment process. For example, ''drug holidays,'' commonly employed with children receiving medication to control hyperactivity, are simply scheduled periods of withdrawal in which the opportunity is presented to evaluate the continued need for intervention. It is not the purpose of withdrawal of the treatment in the BAB design to produce deterioration in a client's performance. The main purpose is to help

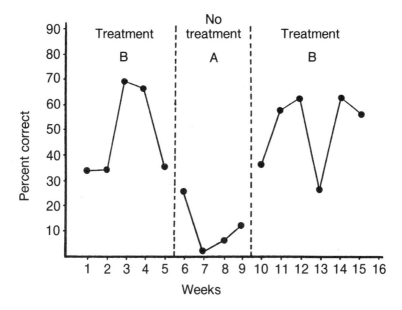

Figure 5.6. Response pattern for a BAB design demonstrating the ability to swallow liquids without loss during periods of oral-motor intervention (B) and a period of no intervention (A).

establish the effectiveness of the intervention and to help determine the need for continued treatment.

Few interventions are such that the treatment can be continued indefinitely. Eventually, there will be a treatment withdrawal or termination; the issue is a matter of timing. Withdrawal employed in the BAB design allows for the assessment of the maintenance of treatment effects. When a temporary cessation of intervention is discussed in this context, few clients or administrators should object.

Changing Criterion Design

Many more complex variations of the AB design are possible. The last design presented in this chapter is the changing criterion design. Additional, more sophisticated design strategies are described in Chapter 6. The changing criterion design is a relatively less frequently appearing design than those previously presented. Yet, for the appropriate situation, the changing criterion design can provide a powerful framework for evaluating clinical change. Kratochwill (1978, p. 66) describes this design as requiring "initial baseline observations on a single behavior. Subsequent to baseline, an intervention program is implemented in each of a series of intervention phases. A stepwise criterion rate for a target behavior is applied during each intervention phase.''

This design is appropriate for use in evaluating clinical change when the goals to be attained in therapy can be broken down into quantifiable successive steps and criteria for change from one step or level to the next can be specified. When these conditions are met, the changing criterion design allows the client to demonstrate sequentially ''higher'' levels of performance. A criterion of successful performance is established during the initial intervention phase. Following successful achievement of this performance level across several trials, or after a stable criterion level is achieved, the criterion is increased. In the next phase, a new and higher level or more difficult criterion is established while the intervention is continued. When behavior or performance reaches this new criterion level and is maintained across trials or time, the next phase, with a more difficult criterion, is introduced. For example, Figure 5.7 graphically demonstrates the progress of a handicapped student in developing independent standing ability (Ottenbacher and York, 1984). In the first phase, the criterion was established as 2 seconds of independent standing. In the second phase, the criterion was increased to 5 seconds of independent standing, and in the third and final phase, the criterion was 10 seconds of independent standing. During each of these phases, the treatment program that the student was receiving to enhance his postural skills remained the same. This procedure is different from the previous designs in which the outcome measure stayed constant but the treatment was manipulated across the design phases (treatment and no-treatment phases). In the changing criterion design, the treatment remains constant across the phases, but the expected outcome or performance level is manipulated or increased across phases. In a sense, the logic of the changing criterion design is slightly different from that applied in other variations of the AB design. The logic of the changing criterion design applies when it is possible to specify or identify the pattern of a given behavior over a particular period and to change the specification for success repeatedly.

A therapist should consider the use of a changing criterion design, instead of use of the simple phase change variations of the AB design described previously, when he or she has some prior expectations regarding the specific pattern of behavior which should be seen. The changing criterion design is most successfully used with behaviors that tend to change gradually in a predictable direction. It is particularly well suited to situations in which the patient is learning a new skill in a gradual pre-determined sequence or is gradually eliminating a problem behavior. It does not require any withdrawal of treatment and, in fact, is logically useful even when no baseline assessment phase is possible.

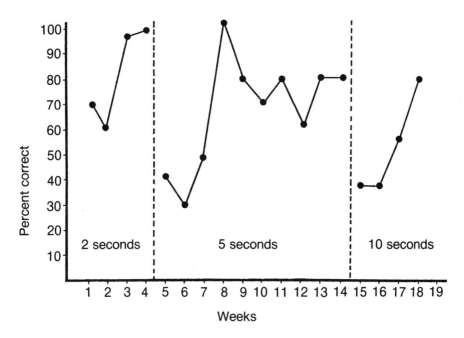

Figure 5.7. Changing criterion design in which the patient demonstrates an increasing ability to stand independently over three phases.

BASIC CONSIDERATIONS RELATED TO DATA COLLECTION

In the previous sections, several basic single system designs are described. These design strategies can form the foundation for evaluating individual change in clinical environments. Before proceeding to the more complex designs presented in the next chapter, it seems appropriate to briefly review some of the fundamental characteristics associated with single system evaluation strategies.

Baseline

As noted earlier, the basic process of the single system framework involves a comparison between data collected when an intervention is in effect and data collected during periods or phases when the intervention is not in effect. A baseline period typically precedes a treatment period, although there is at least one design variation presented in this chapter, the BAB design, that departs from this sequence and includes a no-treatment period between two intervention periods. The importance of a baseline in providing a standard for comparison of treatment efforts during the intervention periods is obvious. Establishing an adequate baseline, however, may be one of the features that the clinician less interested in "research" control may be tempted to eliminate. As Thomas (1979, p. 22) notes, "taking an adequate baseline might delay intervention and also impose on the client an otherwise extraneous measurement task." On the other hand, an adequate baseline provides very useful clinical information to assess both treatment effectiveness and client progress. As noted in a previous section, the securing of baseline data may occur naturally or simultaneously with other pretreatment activities and not adversely affect or delay treatment.

Consistency

The consistency of observation and recording procedures will help ensure that reliable data are collected and that the data accurately represent the client's actual performance level. Hersen (1973, p. 1) states that whenever possible, all measurements should be similar "with respect to measurement devices used, personnel involved, time or times of day measurements are recorded, instructions to the subject, and the specific environmental conditions (i.e., location) where the measurement sessions occur." A therapist would be ill advised to compare, for example, a client's blood pressure and/or heart rate taken prior to therapy during one week with that taken immediately following therapy the next week. Obviously, the therapy sessions could affect these measures, and conclusions drawn from data collected in such a manner would be difficult to interpret. Issues related to accurately and reliably recording client performance, which are discussed in the previous chapter, must be considered in implementing any single system design.

Frequency of Data Collection

As noted previously, repeated collection of data is one of the distinguishing characteristics of single system evaluation strategies. Data should be collected repeatedly over time within each treatment and no-treatment phase. Data collected only before and after intervention (pretest/posttest) would seriously limit the ability to draw conclusions about the effect of the intervention for a single client or a small group of patients. There are no formal rules for the exact frequency of data collection, as this, in part, is determined by the dictates of the particular problem under treatment and the stability of the data (see later discussion of stability). Barlow and Hersen (1973) have argued that at least three data points are needed to determine a trend in the data. Other authorities (Kazdin, 1982) have suggested that six to eight data points per phase be considered a minimum. The need to collect data repeatedly should lead the clinician to select outcome measures related to treatment that occur frequently enough for the therapist to gather the required amount of data in a reasonable period of time.

Alternate measures that are related to the client's problem and are sensitive enough to provide data points may be needed to replace or augment the measurement of rare-occurrence or low-incidence measures (Jayaratne and Levy, 1979). For example, although a problem event such as a heart attack might be quite rare, other events directly related to the problem, such as heart rate and blood pressure, may be recorded on a regular basis. For cases in which extreme rarity is not a problem, frequency of data collection will be determined by the frequency at which the behavior or performance being measured is likely to occur and by the nature of the problem or goal. For instance, if a problem behavior occurs immediately after the client takes a weekly prescribed drug, weekly measurement may be the logical choice. On the other hand, a child's self-abusive behavior may need to be monitored on a daily or even an hourly basis.

Stability

Data within each phase should attain a degree of stability before the therapist moves on to the next design phase, whenever this is possible. A stable data pattern permits clear comparisons across the various conditions or phases. Although stability is the ideal, Kazdin (1978) notes that a trend in one phase opposite to the direction one would expect, based on performance in a previous phase, should not seriously affect the ability to draw inferences about the treatment even when the data are relatively unstable. Trends in the same direction, of course, would affect the ability to draw conclusions from highly unstable data and may indicate the need for statistical procedures to assist in comparing client performance across phases. We have more to say regarding stability of data and data interpretation in later chapters.

CONCLUSION

The characteristic or fundamental form of the within-subject design discussed in previous sections is the AB design, in which A represents the baseline or pretreatment (no-treatment) condition and B represents the intervention phase. Variations of this basic design are the ABA, ABAB, BAB, and so on. The main advantage of these basic within-subject single system strategies is that a functional relationship between the intervention and the outcome measure can be assessed when the treatment procedures are withdrawn and then reinstated. In addition, the designs can demonstrate the progress, or lack of progress, made by specific clients while they are receiving intervention.

The basic designs presented in this chapter constitute the foundation for evaluating client change with use of single system strategies. The designs illustrated are often referred to as within-subject designs, since measurements and treatments are manipulated within one individual (or a small group) across different phases. These basic designs can provide substantial evidence that changes in a client's performance are attributable to the treatment procedures. They also can provide a method of systematically documenting and demonstrating individual client change during the course of intervention. This accountability aspect of these basic designs is one of the strongest arguments for their routine use in clinical environments.

CHAPTER 6

Intermediate and Advanced Designs for Single System Evaluation and Research

INTRODUCTION

In Chapter 5, several basic single system designs are presented which provide the foundation for the systematic evaluation of therapeutic interventions. In this chapter, some additional designs are described. In general, these designs allow the therapist to answer more questions related to the assessment of therapeutic practice. As noted in the introduction to Chapter 5, single system designs can be used as a method of documenting clinical change in individual patients. The strategies can also be used to demonstrate a causal relationship between a treatment and an outcome. Several of the basic designs presented in the previous chapter allow the therapist to document whether a clinically meaningful change in performance has occurred during the period of evaluation. Designs such as the basic AB design, however, do not provide convincing evidence that the treatment employed was causally related to any improvement recorded during the intervention phase. With use of several of the designs presented in this chapter, the therapist can have added confidence in making causal inferences related to the efficacy of treatment.

These designs, including multiple baseline procedures, multiple probe designs, alternating treatment procedures, simultaneous treatment designs and interaction designs, provide the clinician with a variety of strategies appropriate for examining and evaluating complex interventions. All of the designs have strengths and weaknesses. The design strategy ultimately selected by a therapist will obviously depend on the nature of the problem under evaluation and the needs of the client and therapist. Multiple baseline designs offer a flexible method of evaluating treatment effectiveness across subjects, settings, and behaviors. They provide the therapist with built-in replication of the intervention effects and do not require the withdrawal of treatment. Multiple baseline procedures are easily implemented in most clinical environments and are widely used to evaluate the effectiveness of interventions in applied settings. If the purpose of evaluation is to compare two or more treatments, some form of alternating treatment design can be employed. Alternating treatment designs allow the therapist to make empirical judgments about the effectiveness of individual treatments in relation to a nontreatment condition or in relation to other selected interventions. If the therapist wishes to evaluate the effectiveness of a treatment package that involves the concurrent administration of one or more treatment components, the simultaneous treatment design may be the method of choice. Finally, if the therapist requires evaluative information on the additive or combined effects of more than one intervention or on the possible interactive effects of two or more treatments, some form of interaction design may be the most appropriate assessment strategy.

————— MULTIPLE BASELINE DESIGNS —————

Use of the multiple baseline design prevents many of the problems associated with reversal strategies, as a return to baseline conditions need not be included. Instead of use of reversal or withdrawal phases to demonstrate treatment effects, the multiple baseline design introduces the intervention, usually at staggered points in time, across separate baselines. This approach allows the therapist to examine (1) one target behavior or performance area across multiple subjects (multiple baseline design across subjects), (2) multiple target behaviors in one subject (multiple baseline design across behaviors), or (3) one behavior in one subject across multiple settings (multiple baseline design across settings).

In this single system design, the intervention is introduced in the first baseline once a stable response pattern is demonstrated. Interventions in the other baselines begin after a stable response to the intervention has been observed in the preceding baseline or after predetermined intervals have passed. At least two separate baselines are required to demonstrate a therapeutic relationship between intervention and behavior, but confidence that the intervention is truly responsible for behavior change increases as changes are noted across multiple baselines (Kazdin, 1982).

Figure 6.1 illustrates the results associated with a multiple baseline design across subjects which was used to assess the effectiveness of an adaptive cup combined with a program of applied behavior management to teach lip closure to three severely multihandicapped students. These three students exhibited the physical ability to obtain lip closure and were identified by residential staff as problem feeders. During the baseline phase of the design, information related to the ability of each student to maintain lip closure was recorded. The adaptive cup included a small spout, which was inserted into the student's mouth. Duration of lip closure around the

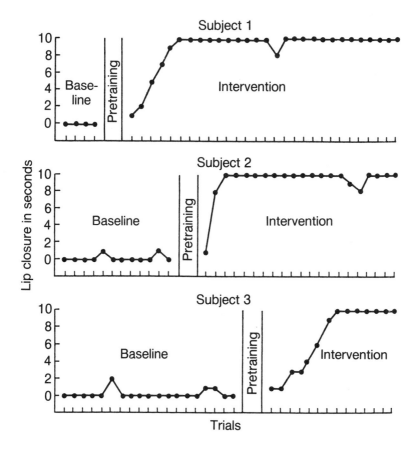

Figure 6.1. Line graph illustrating a multiple baseline design across three subjects.

spout was recorded in seconds (up to a maximum of 10 seconds for each trial). Once a stable level of performance was achieved during baseline, the intervention was administered to each of the three students in a sequentially staggered schedule, and the duration of lip closure per trial was recorded.

The intervention consisted of a shaping procedure in which successive approximations of lip closure were reinforced with delivery of a small amount of liquid by the use of a flow control device mounted on the adaptive cup (see Ottenbacher and York, 1984). The consistently increasing performance of each individual client as the intervention was introduced indicates the effectiveness of the procedure across the different students.

The flexibility of the multiple baseline design may not be immediately apparent and warrants a more detailed examination. First, note that in Figure 6.1, each of the three separate clients (subjects 1, 2 and 3) are dealt with individually with what appears to be an AB design. More importantly, note that the baseline measurement for each student begins at the same time and continues for each student as the intervention is introduced. Second, the interventions used with the second and the third student are identical with the intervention used with the first student. Also, the intervention for the first student does not begin until there is a relatively stable baseline and is not introduced to the second student until a response pattern of significant change has been established for the first student. This set of conditions is repeated for the third student and for however many clients are being included in the evaluation. If, as depicted in Figure 6.1 and described in the earlier example, changes in the expected direction occur during the sequential intervention phase (and only during those periods), there is a logical basis for inferring that the treatment was functionally linked to the desired changes. The effects of extraneous factors, history in particular, have been effectively eliminated. There is a clear correspondence between the changes in the performance of the individual students and the implementation of intervention at different periods of time; the changes come about only after an intervention is introduced.

As noted previously, the same basic multiple baseline procedure may also be used to evaluate the effects of intervention across settings or across behaviors within the same client. It is this flexibility that makes the multiple baseline design such a powerful single system evaluation strategy. In the example just presented, a therapist might be interested in demonstrating that the intervention strategy used to obtain lip closure would be effective for a specific client in multiple settings. A multiple baseline design across settings could be employed to determine the answer to this clinical question in an empirically valid manner. In such a design, the method of recording baseline measures and of delivering the intervention would stay the same. Only one client would be evaluated, however, and the baseline and intervention phases would be conducted in multiple settings. For example, setting 1 might be the clinic where the student receives therapy, setting 2 could be the dining area where the client usually eats his or her meals, and setting 3 might be a snack or lounge area where the student spends leisure time but also is allowed to eat and drink. Figure 6.2 displays a schematic representation of this hypothetical multiple baseline design across settings; various settings in which evaluative information might be collected are indicated. The capability of this particular type of multiple baseline design to demonstrate the generalizability of a therapeutic outcome should be obvious. This generalizability is a vital aspect of documenting treatment effectiveness and is well accomplished with use of the multiple baseline design across settings.

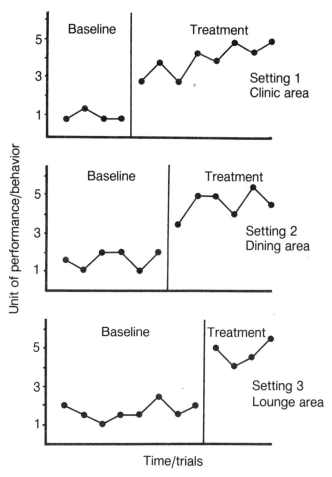

Figure 6.2.   Line graph illustrating a multiple baseline design across three different settings for the same client.

The final version of the multiple baseline design is the application of multiple baselines across behaviors within the same client. In this design strategy, the client, the setting, and the intervention remain the same, but the outcome measures or the behaviors targeted for change are varied. In the previous example, the intervention would remain constant, but the behaviors might be expanded to include other motor skills or postural functions also needed in the feeding process. For instance, in the same client a therapist may use the applied behavioral intervention strategy to facilitate lip closure, head control, and erect trunk posture in sitting.

In the multiple baseline design across behaviors, relatedness or dependency between the selected target behaviors can be a problem. The more interrelated the behaviors, the more likely they are to be immediately influenced when the intervention is applied to any one of them. For example, if the selected behaviors were lip closure, swallowing, and tongue protrusion, the probability is high that as soon as one behavior changes, the other two would also be modified. When the multiple target behaviors or performance areas react at the same time to one intervention, the logical basis for concluding that the intervention is producing a unique effect on the target behavior is markedly reduced.

Another general limitation of the multiple baseline strategy is that it requires the concurrent measurement of performance across several individuals, settings, or behaviors. Thus, it requires more time, more materials and, perhaps, more personnel to implement properly. The multiple baseline designs also require a prolonged baseline condition when the intervention is introduced last. In the previous example of a multiple baseline design across subjects (Figure 6.1), the first student began to receive the intervention after a relatively short baseline of four trials. Due to the requirement that the baselines be staggered, the third student received a much longer baseline and did not begin to receive the intervention until a total of 19 trials had passed. This prolonged baseline period may present some practical difficulties in clinical settings where a long delay in treatment cannot be tolerated. In fact, in this example each of the trials consisted of the presentation of 1½ oz of liquid to the client. Several trials were associated with each meal, so that the total period of baseline, even for subject 3, was less than 5 days.

Watson and Workman (1981) have introduced a version of the multiple baseline design which is intended to address the two limitations referred to previously. They argue that the multiple baseline design across subjects can be subdivided into two distinct design options. One of these options, which is described previously and presented graphically in Figure 6.1, is the traditional multiple baseline design across subjects. Watson and Workman (1981) refer to this option as the *concurrent* multiple baseline design across subjects, which indicates that all subjects included in the evaluation begin the baseline phase concurrently (see Figure 6.1). As noted previously, this can be a limitation in some clinical settings. Watson and Workman (1981, p. 258) accurately state that "the requirement that observations be taken concurrently clearly poses problems for researchers in applied settings (e.g., schools, mental health centers), since clients with the same target behavior may only infrequently be referred at the same point in time." To deal with this difficulty, Watson and Workman (1981) have introduced the *nonconcurrent* multiple baseline design across individuals. This design does not require that all clients included in the evaluation begin the baseline phase at the same time. To implement this particular design, the therapist must select the length for several baseline periods before the evaluation begins. Then these baseline lengths are randomly assigned to clients as they become available for inclusion in the evaluation. For example, suppose a therapist determined, a priori, that three clients would be evaluated and that the length of the baseline phases would be 5, 10, and 15 days. When the first client that meets the criteria for inclusion in the evaluation becomes available, the client is randomly assigned to one of the baseline conditions. When the second client becomes available, he or she is randomly assigned to one of the remaining baseline lengths. The third client is then assigned to the final baseline length. Assume, for the sake of illustration, that this procedure resulted in the first client being assigned the baseline of 10 days, the second client being assigned to the baseline of 15 days, and the third client being assigned to the baseline of 5 days. Baseline measures are carried out for each of the predetermined baseline periods, and if the clients' response patterns are relatively stable, the intervention is introduced at the predetermined time. Measurement and recording are continued throughout the intervention phase, as with the traditional multiple baseline design. Figure 6.3 is a graphic presentation of this nonconcurrent baseline design.

Watson and Workman (1981) suggest that those clients who fail to display a stable response pattern during the predetermined baseline periods should be dropped from the evaluation and replaced by new clients. For those "dropped" individuals evaluation should be continued with use of an AB format, however, since their response patterns might eventually serve as useful replication data.

Barlow and Hersen (1984) state that the nonconcurrent multiple baseline design may be useful when a therapist is unable to obtain concurrent observations for several clients. They argue, however, that the nonconcurrent approach is less desirable than the traditional multiple baseline design across subjects and that it should only be employed when the standard approach is not feasible.

The primary advantage of these multiple baseline designs is that they do not require a reversal or withdrawal of therapeutic procedures in order to

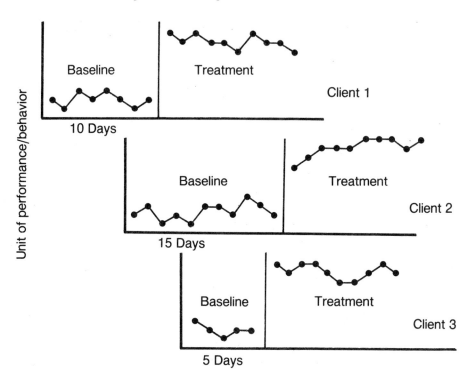

Figure 6.3. Example of a nonconcurrent multiple baseline design across clients. Clients are randomly assigned to predetermined baseline periods (see text for explanation).

provide a convincing demonstration of treatment effectiveness. This feature has several obvious advantages. First, many behaviors or skills acquired in clinical environments are functionally irreversible (Cuvo, 1979). Second, some applications of designs requiring a withdrawal or temporary termination of the treatment may be considered ethically inappropriate, especially if the behavior or performance gains cannot be easily reinstated after a withdrawal of treatment and reduction or leveling off of performance (Murphy and Bryan, 1980). Lastly, some therapists and practitioners unfamiliar with the requirements and value of temporary treatment withdrawals may object to any requirement to interrupt or stop therapy.

One additional advantage of multiple baseline procedures is that they require the concurrent measurement across several behaviors, settings, or subjects. Earlier, this feature was described as a limitation because it generally means that more time, effort and resources will have to be devoted to implementing multiple baseline designs. This is a legitimate limitation. The additional measurement required in multiple behaviors, settings, or subjects, however, is also an advantage. Essentially, each subject, behavior, or setting is providing an opportunity to replicate the effects found in the previous subject, setting, or behavior. This built-in replication provides a degree of generalizability for the results of multiple baseline designs which is not found in other within-subject single system designs. In a later chapter, we have more to say about the issue of generalizability and its importance. For now, it is sufficient to note that the opportunity for generalization is an important advantage associated with multiple baseline procedures.

Multiple Probe Designs

The multiple probe procedure is a variation of the multiple baseline design (Horner and Baer, 1978). The multiple probe design is similar to the multiple baseline design in that the intervention is sequentially introduced across the multiple baselines of subjects, settings, or behaviors. Unlike the multiple baseline design in which the outcome measure is continuously recorded across the various settings, behaviors, or subjects for each phase, however, performance in the multiple probe design is recorded intermittently by the use of "probes." The probe trials are interspersed within the phases of the design and provide the therapist with information that can be used to evaluate the client's level of performance prior to treatment and whether performance improves once the intervention is introduced. The multiple probe design is particularly useful when a therapist is teaching a sequence of steps similar to those frequently followed in task analysis. In this procedure, the therapist first determines the sequence by which a particular skill or task is to be acquired, then introduces the intervention sequentially across the steps after the client has demonstrated mastery of prerequisite skills. Using the multiple probe design, the therapist introduces probes, or intermittent measurements, during or before the first few sessions in which any particular step in the skill sequence is to be acquired. Thus, the therapist can determine whether the intervention exerted an effect at different times (probes). When the multiple probe design is used in this manner, there are as many demonstrations of effectiveness, or lack of effectiveness, as there are steps in the acquisition of the skill.

A note of caution is required regarding the use of multiple probe designs in which intermittent and interspersed problems are conducted. When using intermittent probes rather than consecutive recording of performance, a therapist needs to collect at least three probe data points on each behavior, or with each subject, or in each setting, prior to introducing the intervention. Tawney and Gast (1984) argue that this represents the minimum number of probes necessary to estimate a trend in performance which can then be used as a standard of comparison for demonstrating the effectiveness of an intervention. They recommend going beyond this minimum requirement and attempting to include five or more probes during a particular phase.

An example may help to clarify the difference between the multiple probe design and the conventional multiple baseline procedure. In the previous example of a multiple baseline design across behaviors, the intervention consisted of a program of response shaping used in conjunction with a reinforcement of a preferred liquid to teach specific motor behaviors related to feeding. In the example, the three separate behaviors being evaluated were lip closure, head control, and erect trunk stability. Each was measured in terms of duration that the behavior could be maintained over a specified interval. Figure 6.4 represents a multiple probe design applied to this particular treatment evaluation. Note that the outcome measures are not recorded continuously across each of the three behaviors. Instead, intermittent probes are administered during various

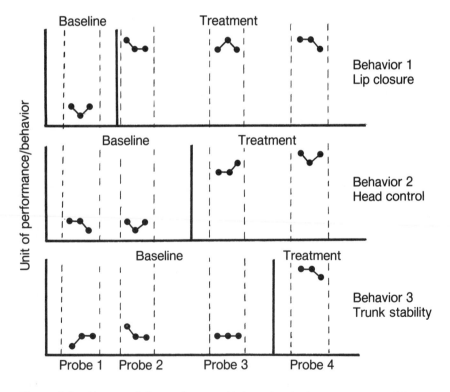

Figure 6.4. Line graph illustrating a multiple probe design across three different behaviors in the same client.

phases of the design. The probes provide information concerning the client's function throughout each of the phases.

The multiple probe design may provide a functional alternative to more conventional multiple baseline procedures. The main advantage of the multiple probe design is that it eliminates the need for a prolonged continuous recording of baseline data. Continuous recording of baseline responses can be time consuming and inconvenient for practicing therapists. The multiple probe strategy allows the intermittent recording of performance and can provide an adequate demonstration of baseline stability, particularly when the behavior being recorded occurs at a low level or there is little chance for the client to "spontaneously" improve. As Cuvo (1979, p. 222) notes, "minimal testing is especially reasonable when the baseline level is low or when there is no opportunity for subjects to acquire the target response(s) without direct training."

Noonan (1984) recently reported on a study evaluating the effectiveness of neuromotor intervention to improve the postural reactions of children with neuromotor disorders. The study employed a multiple baseline design across subjects. Several postural reactions, including the asymmetrical tonic neck reflex (ATNR), the ability to maintain the head erect, and rolling, were measured. These three dependent variables were assessed with use of a multiple probe approach. Noonan (1984, p. 113) states that "the ATNR and head erect or rolling were probed rather than measured each session to reduce the possibility of reactive effects for repeated measurement."

Obviously, that fewer responses are recorded during baseline probe periods can be a disadvantage in some cases. This is a particular limitation in those instances in which there is considerable variability in the response pattern. The intermittent probes may not provide enough information to adequately evaluate the effects of response variability on the client's performance. If there appears to be a significant degree of variability in the client's responses, the therapist may need to extend the baseline period so that more probes can be taken. If adequate stability is not achieved, an alternative design may be indicated.

As noted previously, a relationship or dependency among behaviors is a particular problem for multiple baseline designs implemented across behaviors. This is also true for multiple probe designs across behaviors. If the behaviors are related, training or therapy directed at one behavior may result in improved performance in the other behaviors. In such a case, intermittent probes may be adversely affected by generalization of improved performance across the behaviors. Although a continuous recording of baseline responses would alert the therapist to the existence of a correlation among the behaviors, this may be more difficult to detect in a multiple probe design. Thus, the therapist using the multiple probe design across behaviors should make a concerted effort to ensure that the behaviors or areas of performance targeted for intervention are functionally independent.

_____ ALTERNATING TREATMENT DESIGN _____

Despite its efficiency and flexibility, the alternating treatment design is reported on infrequently in the rehabilitation literature. This design is particularly well suited to comparison of the relative merits of two treatments or different versions of the same treatment. It can also be used, however, to compare treatment versus no-treatment conditions (Barlow and Hayes, 1979). Variations of this design have been referred to in the literature as multiple schedule design (Leitenberg, 1973), a randomized design (Edington, 1980), a multielement design (Sulzer-Azaroff and Mayer, 1977), and a simultaneous treatment design (Kazdin and Hartman, 1978). With the alternating treatment design, the subject is exposed to baseline and alternating treatment conditions throughout the evaluation period; each phase is usually of short duration. A baseline period is not an absolute requirement for an alternating treatment design, although it is very useful. In the alternating treatment design, the baseline both allows a description of initial client function and provides a basis for prediction of the future course of performance. If an alternating treatment design is used with only two or more intervention conditions, some assessment of the impact of the treatment per se as well as differential treatment effects is allowed. If a baseline is included, a more informative comparison is possible. One of the few examples of an alternating treatment design in the recent physical and occupational therapy literature is provided by Ottenbacher and York (1984). With this design, the effects of three different forms of intervention related to improving the self-feeding skills of a student with mental retardation were compared. The design is presented in Figure 6.5. The first phase (B) displays the percent correct responses for self-feeding. The treatment administered during this phase included physical assistance from the teacher in orienting and guiding the spoon from a standard compartmentalized lunch tray to the client's mouth. In phase C, the use of physical assistance to guide the student's movements was eliminated, and the intervention consisted only of verbal cues and directions to the student regarding his self-feeding. Finally, in the third phase of the design (D), the intervention involved substituting the use of a scoop dish in place of the standard lunch tray. No verbal or physical assistance was provided during the last phase. The graphic evidence presented in the figure clearly indicates a difference in response patterns across the alternating forms of intervention. This design represents a very basic example of the

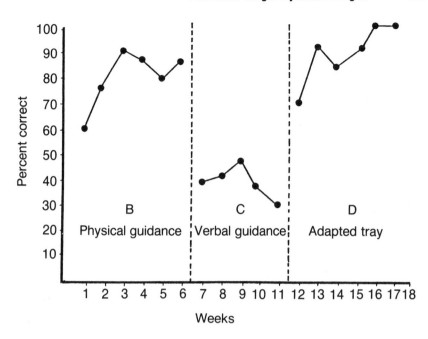

Figure 6.5. Line graph illustrating an alternating treatment design. Response patterns for three different treatments are compared across the three phases.

alternating treatment design in which three different interventions are varied or alternated for a single client. The results provide systematic documentation of the client's responses during each of the design phases, but the design provides little evidence of a functional or causal relationship between the treatments and the client's responses.

More sophisticated applications of the alternating treatment design are possible, particularly when the opportunity for several alterations of the treatment are available. Suppose, for example, that the goal of a therapy team was to reduce the incidence of self-stimulating behavior in a child who was diagnosed as autistic. For illustrative purposes, assume that an appropriate procedure for recording the number or amount of self-stimulating behaviors has been developed. This might consist of a partial time sample during which the number of self-stimulating behaviors are recorded for a predetermined period of time. Let us assume also that the occurrence of a self-stimulating behavior has been operationally defined. In this example, an alternating treatment design is used to compare the effects of two separate interventions to each other and to a baseline. The first intervention consists of 45 minutes of sensory integrative activities individually designed and administered to the subject. The sensory integrative treatment includes planned activities selected to provide various amounts of tactile, proprioceptive, and vestibular stimulation designed to enhance the child's sensory processing ability and facilitate adaptive behavior. The second treatment includes 45 minutes of "pet" therapy in which the child is exposed to various animals and encouraged to interact with them in an appropriate manner. Each of the therapies are administered by a competently trained specialist familiar with the intervention procedures. The recording of self-stimulatory behavior occurs during a half-hour period immediately following the therapy sessions. Finally, the baseline period consists of time spent in the school classroom on a standard school program. For the requirements of the design to be met, each therapy is provided for only a 2-day period before the switch is made to the next phase.

Figure 6.6 displays the hypothetical outcome of this design. The A phases represent baseline periods during which the child took part in the standard school activities and self-stimulating behaviors were monitored during a predetermined half-hour period each day. The B phases represent those days when the child received sensory integrative therapy, and the C phases represent those periods when the child received the program of pet therapy. In this hypothetical example of the alternating treatment design, only two data points are collected during each phase before the next

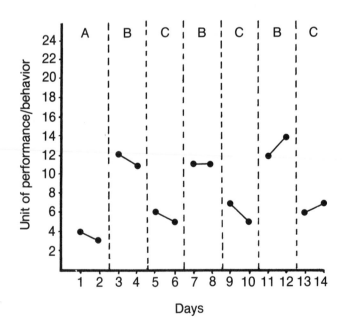

Figure 6.6. Data points for individual phases in an alternating treatment design. See the text for a description of the treatment associated with each phase.

intervention or phase in introduced. Because of the rapid alteration of phases, there is no opportunity to establish the stability or trend of performance within any given phase. Rather, these assessments are obtained within conditions by collapsing or arranging data points for each condition or treatment into a separate series. That is, all the data points for the A phase are plotted in series, as are all the data points for each of the treatment conditions (phases B and C). Figure 6.7 displays the plotted data points collapsed for each of the respective conditions. If there is a clear separation between the series of data points, a difference in performance among the conditions may be inferred.

The previous example of the alternating treatment design provides a hypothetical illustration of how the design can be used to provide empirical comparisons between treatments for the same disorder. In many areas, practitioners are often forced to choose between two closely related types of treatments or interventions for the same dysfunction. For example, a therapist may be exposed to conflicting views about the best way to manage upper extremity spasticity in a patient who has suffered a cerebrovascular accident (CVA). Arguments may be made that splinting with a volar resting hand splint is most appropriate, while counterarguments that a dorsal resting hand splint is the preferred method may appear just as valid. Distinctions between two related treatments are extremely difficult to make

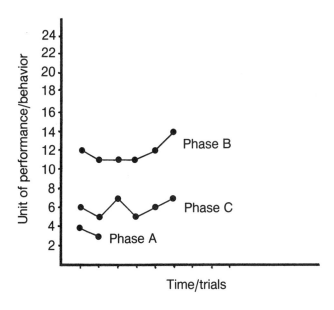

Figure 6.7. Response patterns collapsed across each phase for the data presented in Figure 6.6.

on a case-by-case basis and are often made by relying on tradition or theoretical logic (Nelson and Hayes, 1979). The therapist familiar with the alternating treatment design can easily develop an effective evaluation strategy that will provide empirical information on which to make these difficult treatment decisions in a way that is individually tailored to the client receiving services.

As previously noted, the alternating treatment design could be conducted without the presence of a baseline. This does not mean that information on pretreatment performance cannot be collected. A variation of the alternating treatment design could be developed in which a pretreatment and posttreatment measure of client performance was recorded across a series of intervention phases. The data points from the phases can then be plotted in series to compare pretreatment (nontreatment) with performance during intervention. For example, a therapist may be interested in the effectiveness of two therapy strategies for improving the perceptual function of a stroke patient who evidences unilateral neglect. One treatment program may be neurophysiologically based and include activities such as brushing, vibration, and related stimulation procedures associated with therapeutic principles developed by Margaret Rood (Trombly, 1982). The second treatment approach may be based on cognitive learning theory and include learning-oriented activities designed to make the client aware of body parts and body and/or spatial relations. The goal of this treatment approach is to teach the patient functional strategies to compensate for perceptual deficits. For this design to be effective, the therapist needs a quick reliable measure of perceptual function appropriate for use with adult clients who have suffered a CVA. The therapist might select the line bisection test developed by Schenkenberg et al. (1980). This test requires the client to bisect a series of horizontal lines and has been shown to be a useful perceptual measure in adults and appropriate for use with brain-injured patients (Van Deusen, 1983). The test is simple to complete and can be administered in a matter of minutes. In the hypothetical design the therapist would administer the line bisection test to the client both immediately before and immediately after each therapy session.

Figure 6.8 depicts the possible outcome of such a design. Each B phase represents a period of intervention in which the neurophysiological treatment procedure was used, and each C phase represents a period of intervention in which the cognitive learning approach was used. In Figure 6.9, the response patterns for the separate phases, including both the preintervention and the postintervention performance, are displayed. Figure 6.9 indicates that both treatments produced an immediate (posttest) improvement in performance relative to the pretest level of performance, but the cognitive learning intervention produced a pattern of lower scores, which indicates better performance on the test than did the neuro-

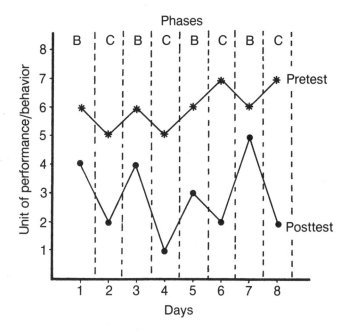

Figure 6.8. Line graph of a pretest and a posttest response pattern for an alternating treatment design.

physiological intervention for this particular client. This design allows a comparison between treatment and no-treatment conditions, even though a baseline phase is not part of the formal design structure. The flexibility of the design is further illustrated by the briefness of the phases. It would be possible to have each alternating phase represent a treatment period of 1 day. These are certainly advantages which make this type of design, or a variation, very compatible with use in most clinical settings.

One advantage of alternating treatment designs is that they do not require a withdrawal of termination of the treatment. If a cessation of intervention is included in the design, it does not need to be very long. If the question under investigation is which of two therapies is most effective, the answer can be provided without any withdrawal of treatment, as was illustrated in the previous examples. A second advantage of the alternating treatment strategy is that the individual phases can be very short in duration and meaningful comparisons can usually be made in a briefer period of time than that required with traditional designs. More conventional designs with fewer phases, such as the ABA, will require the phases to be long enough to produce stable response patterns and also require a withdrawal. Since data points in most alternating treatment designs are taken across a series of

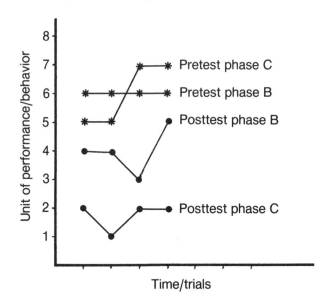

Figure 6.9. Line graph illustrating response patterns collapsed across phases for pretest and posttest conditions depicted in Figure 6.8.

phases spread over the entire design, fewer data points may be required. This is because assessment of variability in an alternating treatment design is inferred, in part, from all of the data, not just those data points within a single phase or a single series. For example, Storey et al. (1984) recently provided an example of the use of an alternating treatment design in a therapy setting. A program of sensory stimulation involving tactile, olfactory, and gustatory input was alternated with nontreatment to reduce self-stimulatory behaviors in a 12-year-old girl with profound mental retardation. Storey et al. (1984, p. 511) state that the ''advantages of this design are that it does not include a withdrawal of treatment and that the comparison may be made more quickly than in a withdrawal design.''

Another major advantage of the alternating treatment design is that it does not require a formal baseline phase. This possibility of implementing the design without a separate baseline phase is a distinct advantage in many clinical settings where therapists may be unable or unwilling to gather baseline information. As noted previously, however, the inclusion of a baseline can strengthen the conclusions drawn from alternating treatment designs, and baselines should be included in the design when this is feasible.

The number of alterations of the phases included in the design is a factor that contributes to the strength of the alternating treatment designs. In general, the more frequent and greater the number of phase alterations, the more opportunity there will be for the series of data points to diverge or overlap. Since the basic comparison in an alternating treatment design is the amount or degree of divergence or overlap between the different series of data points for each condition, an increase in the frequency and number of phase alterations increases the precision of the analysis and the strength of the design. Of course, there are several limitations related to the alterations included in an alternate treatment design. Often these limitations are related to the meaningfulness of the measurement unit. The measurement frequency and measurement unit should be dictated by the needs of the client and the nature of the problem, not by the design.

The primary disadvantage or limitation associated with an alternating treatment design is the possibility of multiple treatment interference. Multiple treatment interference refers to the fact that the two or more treatments being evaluated may interact in some fashion to produce an effect that would not be present if any treatment were applied in isolation. In other words, the results of treatment X may not be the same when it is applied by itself as when it precedes or follows treatment Y in an alternating treatment design.

The effects of multiple ''interventions'' is an issue with which therapists are familiar. Clients receiving therapy are continuously exposed to a number of factors which influence their response to particular treatments. A television program the client saw the night before, the argument he had with his son earlier in the day, or a multitude of other events might influence how he or she performs in the clinical setting. With the alternating treatment design, an attempt is made to determine the extent to which two or more interventions affect client performance. Obviously, there is the possibility that these interventions will interact and affect client performance in a complicated fashion. Barlow and Hayes (1979) have identified two possible confounds related to multiple treatment inference. They include sequencing or order effects and carryover effects.

Sequencing or order effects refer to the fact that when multiple treatments are provided in a particular order, behavior changes could be a function of prior treatments interacting with a treatment that is currently being provided. Order effects are not unique to alternating treatment designs; they also occur in group-comparison procedures in which two or more treatments are employed. Sequencing or order effects are typically controlled by counterbalancing the interventions. Counter-balancing of the interventions can control for order effects resulting from one treatment always preceding or following another. Counterbalancing also helps control for extraneous variables that might affect performance. These variables might include the time of day the intervention is provided, the therapist who is treating the client, or the setting in which the intervention is administered. For example, if treatment X is always administered by the physical therapist and treatment Y is always administered by the occupational therapist, it would be difficult to isolate the effect of the treatment from the different therapists. It is possible that the more effective treatment was successful because of some undefined characteristic of the therapist administering that particular intervention rather than because of the treatment itself. By counterbalancing the design so that the physical therapist administers both treatments and the occupational therapist also administers treatment X on one day and treatment Y on another day, the effects of the different therapists can be spread equally across both treatments and, therefore, neutralized. Counterbalancing of treatments, therapists, time of treatment administrations, and settings allows for control of these possible confounding variables and permits the therapist to have additional confidence that outcomes are functionally related to specific interventions. Table 6.1 presents an example of a design for counterbalancing two treatments, A and B, administered by two therapists, Jane and John. Note, in the table, that not only do Jane and John administer both treatments but the order is also counterbalanced so that one treatment is not always presented before the other.

Through alternating and counterbalancing, the effect of a particular therapist is controlled. The treatments are presented in a random order to prevent development of a pattern for treatment presentations; the alternating treatment design requires that the treatments be administered an equal number of times, however. In Table 6.1, notice that both treatments A and B are presented an equal number of times (8) and that Jane and John administer each of the treatments an equal number of times. The design is thus balanced for treatment order and for the influence of the two therapists.

This design represents a fairly simple example of counterbalancing. For example, a therapist may wish to counterbalance for effects due to time of day and setting, among other factors. In such a case the process of counterbalancing becomes more complex. Therapists should keep in mind that the more treatments included in the design the more complex the design becomes in terms of possible multiple treatment effects. Kazdin and Hartman (1978) recommend that with use of an alternating treatment design no more than two or three treatments be compared in one evaluation attempt; otherwise, the design becomes too complicated to implement in typical applied or clinical environments.

Carryover effects are the second possible confound that may effect the results of an alternating treatment design and limit the confidence a therapist might have in establishing a functional relationship between the treatment and the client's performance. Carryover effects refer to the influence on the adjacent treatment, regardless of the overall sequencing.

Table 6.1.
Example of Counterbalancing of Treatments A and B for Two Different
Therapists

Trials	Therapist	Treatment
1	Jane	A
2	John	B
3	Jane	B
4	John	A
5	Jane	B
6	John	A
7	Jane	A
8	John	B
9	Jane	B
10	John	A
11	Jane	B
12	John	A
13	Jane	A
14	John	B
15	Jane	A
16	John	B

The distinction between carryover effects and sequencing effects is a subtle one (Kratochwill and Levin, 1980). The difference is often defined in terms of the extent of the effect. In sequencing or order effects, each treatment in a sequence may cumulatively affect subsequent treatments. For instance, treatment A may influence treatment B, and treatments A and B may affect treatment C, and so on. Carryover effects, on the other hand, are more localized and are analyzed in terms of adjacent phases or interventions only. Ulman and Sulzer-Azaroff (1975) divide carryover effects into two categories: contrast and induction. In contrast carryover effects, the performance in the two conditions associated with the two treatments change in opposite directions. In other words, if performance on the outcome measure increases when treatment B is administered, it will decrease when treatment C is administered. With induction carryover effects, the performance change is in the same direction for both of the treatments, and the effect of the first treatment may be facilitory to the second treatment.

Therapists employing alternating treatment designs should be aware of the possibility of carryover effects. If there is the potential for either type of carryover effect, the therapist should take this into account and qualify the results of the evaluation accordingly.

There are several possible ways to reduce carryover effects, which include counterbalancing, the use of short treatment phases and providing a separation between the treatment periods (Sidman, 1960). Empirically, the impact of carryover effects has been shown to be minimal (Ulman and Sulzer-Azaroff, 1975), and investigators using alternating treatment designs often do not attempt to control for them.

SIMULTANEOUS TREATMENT AND INTERACTION DESIGNS

Simultaneous treatment designs and interaction designs represent expansions of the alternating treatment design discussed in the previous section. These designs are generally more complex and sophisticated than the alternating treatment designs. Because of their increased complexity they may provide the therapist with more information in assessing a functional relationship between a treatment and a particular patient outcome. The interaction designs allow the therapist to answer more questions related to the effects of the treatment, particularly as they are related to other treatments or combinations of treatment. On the negative side, the complexity of these designs often limits their usefulness in clinical environments. They are infrequently used in applied settings where they may be very difficult to implement. Consequently, they will be only briefly presented here.

As noted in the previous section, the effects of multiple treatments can be compared with use of the alternating treatment designs. One of the distinguishing characteristics of the alternating treatment design is that the treatments are presented or administered sequentially in an alternating or counterbalanced fashion. The important distinction between alternating treatment designs and simultaneous treatment designs is that in the latter the treatments are administered simultaneously in one phase. The schematic for such a design may appear as A BC A CB, in which B and C represent two different treatments administered during the same phase. In a simultaneous treatment design the treatments are available simultaneously. The client is administered a combination of both treatments or is allowed to choose which intervention will be applied.

If the client is given a choice between two simultaneously presented interventions, the primary purpose of the design is to assess client preference for a particular form of intervention. This application of the simultaneous treatment design is more likely to be found in studies of applied behavioral management in which a client may be presented with a choice between a verbal or edible reinforcement or some similar arrangement of contingencies. This application of the design has a limited relevance to most settings in which occupational and physical therapists will be evaluating client performance. If the two treatments are presented in combination and the client receives both interventions simultaneously, the purpose of the design is to assess the effectiveness of a combination of the two treatments. For example, suppose a therapist used two treatment strategies to help reduce the extraneous movements in the upper extremities of a client diagnosed as having athetoid cerebal palsy. Assume that the outcome measure of interest in the evaluation was the ability to communicate by use of a specially adapted typewriter. Due to the client's athetoid movements, however, he is unable to use the typewriter in an efficient manner. One "treatment" might consist of placing a weighted wrist cuff on the client's right upper extremity. The second "treatment" might consist of having the client grasp an upright dowel secured to a table top or other surface with his left hand. The purpose of grasping the dowel with the left upper extremity would be to stabilize the left arm and reduce the incidence of associated movements. A combination of these "treatments" may be effective in reducing the presence of athetoid movements in the right upper extremity and, thereby, increase the efficiency of the client's typing.

The simultaneous treatment design permits an analysis of the effects of several interventions implemented concurrently. Because of its rather narrow focus in establishing treatment efficacy, it is not well suited for the general evaluation of treatment outcome.

A more clinically relevant design may be achieved by combining aspects of the alternating treatment design and simultaneous treatment design into what is referred to as an interaction design. The purpose of an interaction design is to evaluate additive, subtractive, and interactive effects of individual treatment components rather that to provide a simple comparison of two or more treatments.

In the typical interaction design the therapist is interested in determining the effects of treatment B and treatment C administered separately and the interactive effects of treatments B and C administered jointly. Thus, each treatment of interest is evaluated alone and in conjunction with other treatments. For instance, in the example presented above, the treatments of interest were the effects of a weighted wrist cuff (treatment B) and stabilization of the contralateral arm (treatment C) to reduce athetoid movements in a client with cerebral palsy who was learning one-handed typing. If the therapist was interested in the interactive effect of these treatments, the following design might be employed A B BC B BC. This design would specifically separate the contributions of the weighted wrist cuff (treatment B) from the interactive effects of both treatments. The A and final BC phase are not essential to the design but follow the conventional format and strengthen the conclusions that can be drawn from the design. The initial baseline is particularly useful in establishing a standard for comparison.

When an interaction design is used in an evaluation, keep the "one variable" rule in mind; i.e., only one variable or treatment can be manipulated at a time in any interaction design. Also, each treatment must be adjacent to one of the treatments against which it is being evaluated. Thus an A BC A B design would not be suitable for evaluating the effectiveness of treatment B and its interaction with treatment C. This is because an intervening A phase appears between the two treatment phases. Unless the treatment components are in adjacent phases and in the appropriate sequence, the therapist cannot adequately evaluate the additive or subtractive effects of the treatments or any possible treatment interactions that may result (Hersen and Barlow, 1976). The true interactive design goes beyond the analysis of separate effects or comparisons of one treatment over a baseline as in A B A C design. Clinical investigators who attempt to use an A B A C design to evaluate additive or combined effects of treatments neglect to consider possible confounds due to ordering or sequencing effects. Even if counterbalancing is introduced in such a design, it is not possible to draw conclusions concerning the effectiveness of the combination of the two treatments because the two have never been combined to determine whether the combination produced effects that are different from those produced in sequence. The effects of treatments B and C can be compared relative to the baseline (A) and to each other, but the combined or interactive effects cannot be determined. Confusion over this and related issues is reflected in the inconsistency in labeling of many advanced single system designs. These designs have been referred to as multielement, multischedule, multitreatment, simultaneous treatment, concurrent treatment, or concurrent schedule. The distinction between these designs and various types of interaction designs is not always clear.

The true interaction design allows the therapist to evaluate the additive, subtractive, and interactive effects of two or more interventions within the design framework. This is accomplished by examining the effect of a treatment alone and in combination with other interventions. When this type of single system design is used, it is possible to evaluate more than two interventions; it is usually not practical to do so, however, since the design becomes complex and very difficult to implement. For example, for exploration of the combined and interactive effects of three treatments, the following inactive design could be used: A B BCD B BCD; C BCD C BCD; D BCD D BCD. Clearly, such a design would present numerous problems in terms of actual implementation in most clinical settings. This design could provide useful data concerning the relative impact of the three treatments and possible interactive and combined effects. If this is the type of information that is desired, the interaction design is certainly appropriate. Obviously, it will require considerable planning and resources to implement such a design successfully. On the other hand, if the therapist is interested only in the overall effects of the combined treatment package, a more straightforward simultaneous treatment design such as A BCD A

BCD would be adequate. This design would allow the therapist to make judgments about the effectiveness of the overall treatment package but would not allow the therapist to attribute treatment effects to specific components of the treatment program.

The primary advantage of the interaction design is that it provides the therapist with valuable information related to the additive, subtractive, and interactive effects of a particular treatment with other interventions and/or factors. In complex clinical situations in which multiple factors influence treatment outcome, this can be very important, particularly if the therapist is interested in larger issues beyond the documentation of client progress, such as validating or refining a knowledge base or theoretical framework. Other advantages of interaction designs are that treatment does not have to be withdrawn and that baseline is not required.

The major disadvantage of interaction designs is that they are complex, sophisticated forms of single system evaluation. Conducting evaluations that employ interaction designs requires a considerable degree of planning and preparation in addition to requiring, generally, more resources and time. Because of these factors, interaction designs are seldom employed in applied settings. There are few examples of these designs even in the applied literature in clinical psychology and special education in which single system approaches have been used extensively. Their infrequent use should not discourage therapists from employing these designs when treatment programs being evaluated require or demand the application of a sophisticated single system approach capable of answering complex questions related to combined or interactive treatment effects.

CONCLUSION

Assessment of complex treatment procedures is a legitimate aspect of evaluation in occupational and physical therapy intervention. As the number and sophistication of the treatment procedures employed by therapists increase, the need for effective methods that provide systematic comparisons between treatments assumes a higher priority.

The designs presented in this chapter, including the multiple baseline design, the multiple probe design, the alternating treatment design, and the simultaneous treatment and interaction design, allow for an in-depth evaluation of various treatment components. As the complexity of the design increases, however, the therapist must be aware of the need to counterbalance and to control for sequencing and order effects. As noted previously, practical consideration may limit the use of some of these designs. Many therapists will decide that the requirements of the advanced designs cannot be met in their particular situations and will rely on the more fundamental single system approaches, presented earlier, to document the effects of intervention. Other therapists may wish to go beyond the simple documentation of clinical change and attempt to demonstrate functional or causal relationships between treatments and client performance or to explore the relative effectiveness of multifaceted treatment procedures in a systematic manner. Clinicians wishing to accomplish these therapeutic goals will require the use of more advanced single system procedures, such as those described in this chapter. The use of these designs and the reporting of the results will help establish a scientific basis for the effectiveness of therapeutic intervention and will help answer complex treatment questions that cannot be resolved by the more basic single system procedures used to document clinical change.

CHAPTER 7

Visual Analysis of Single System Data

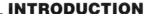

INTRODUCTION

Previous chapters include detailed information on a number of issues related to implementing single system evaluation strategies. The parameters discussed include the importance of measurement and recording procedures and the characteristics of various designs appropriate for evaluating change in individual consumers of therapy services. Obviously, familiarity with only measurement and recording procedures or design strategies will not provide the therapist with all the necessary skills to identify functional relationships between various treatments and outcomes of therapeutic interest. Once the outcome behavior has been identified, the appropriate design has been selected, and the data have been collected, the data are analyzed. Evaluation of the data includes a discussion and a description of the methods used to interpret and draw conclusions about changes of the client's performance or behavior. Graphic presentation and visual analysis have been the traditional methods used with single system designs. According to Kazdin (1982, p. 232), visual inspection "refers to reaching a judgment about the reliability or consistency of intervention effects by visually examining graphed data." Visual inspection involves judging the extent to which changes in response patterns for a particular client are evident across phases within a design and whether the changes are consistent with the requirements of the particular design.

As noted in previous chapters, one of the distinguishing characteristics of single system evaluation strategies is the repeated measurement of client performance over time. The effects of a particular intervention are evaluated at different times, and visual inspection allows the therapist to make judgments based on the overall pattern of data.

The effect of a particular intervention is apparent when systematic changes in performance occur during each phase in which the treatment is present or absent. Similarly, in multiple baseline designs, the intervention is sequentially replicated across individuals, settings or behaviors, and changes in response patterns are visually assessed across these dimensions. Tawney and Gast (1984) argue that graphic presentation and visual inspection of single system data can furnish practitioners with a compact and detailed account of client performance that provides a sequence of the various phases, an indication of the time spent in each phase, and the relationship between the treatment and outcome variables.

In addition, relying on visual inspection of the data predisposes the analysis to detection of clinically important treatment effects. Generally, in visual examination of data from single system designs, changes in response patterns across the various phases must be large enough to allow no room for ambiguous interpretation of treatment effects. Parsonson and Baer (1978) argue that if the treatment effects are so weak that they cannot readily be detected by visual inspection, they are probably equally weak clinically and, therefore, of questionable value in terms of use in clinical environments. For example, Kazdin (1977) contends that a reduction in self-injurious behavior in an autistic child from 80% to 40% is not a clinically significant treatment effect. To obtain a therapeutically significant effect would require a reduction in self-injurious behavior to a near 0% level. Only at this level would the child be considered to no longer require intervention. Traditionally, the underlying rationale for the use of graphic analysis and visual inspection has been that therapists should seek only those treatments that produce large treatment effects and that such effects should be obvious from visual inspection of the data (Baer, 1977; Michael, 1974). This rationale has been challenged in recent years, and a wider variety of analytical methods are now available to evaluate single system data. These alternative methods and some of the advantages and disadvantages of graphic analysis and visual inspection are presented later in this chapter.

Graphic analysis and visual inspection remain the most widely used and easily understood methods of data analysis for single system designs, and therapists evaluating individual clinical change need to be familiar with these techniques. The basic methods and procedures associated with graphic analysis are presented next.

GRAPHIC ANALYSIS

Information presented in previous chapters emphasizes the importance of maintaining systematic records of client performance and developing design strategies that provide data on the effect of particular interventions. By using these procedures, therapists can generate information that will allow them (1) to compare the client's behavior or performance across design phases, (2) to compare differential effects of treatments, and (3) to determine the magnitude of behavioral change. Graphic presentation of data is a convenient method which provides a visual comparison by clients, colleagues, and administrators or supervisors.

Standard graphic arrangements employ two axes drawn at right angles. The horizontal axis or x-axis usually is divided according to units of time (minutes, hours, days, etc.) or trials, while the vertical axis or y-axis contains units of measurement related to frequency, rate, amount, duration, etc., of client behavior (see Figure 7.1).

Simple Line Graph

The simplest form of graphic presentation used with single system designs is the noncumulative or simple line graph. For construction of a simple line graph, client responses are plotted on squared graph paper. The

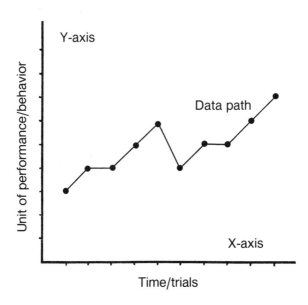

Figure 7.1. Components of typical graph, including y-axis and x-axis.

amount of behavior (y-axis) is plotted at the intersection of the time section (x-axis). After data points have been plotted, they are connected to form a data path. For example, suppose a client with a heart condition is referred for an exercise program to help reduce his weight. The graph depicted in Figure 7.2 illustrates the outcome of this hypothetical treatment program in which a simple AB design is used. The client's ''performance,'' in this case weight in pounds (y-axis), is plotted over time measured in weeks (x-axis). A variation of this graph will provide a good example which can be expanded in the next section to provide an illustration of a cumulative graph. For a simple line graph, the data for the client are plotted each week (day, hour, etc.) in a noncumulative fashion. Figure 7.2 depicts the number of pounds the client lost or gained on a weekly basis. The number of pounds are recorded in relation to the client's weight for the week immediately prior (the client is only weighed once a week).

As a method of data presentation, the simple line graph depicted in Figure 7.2 has several advantages. The graphing technique is familiar and widely recognized by clinicians; thus it is easily interpreted and understood. Simple line graphs are easy to construct and permit the continuous monitoring and evaluation of client performance. Such information makes it easier for the therapist to know when to modify or terminate intervention.

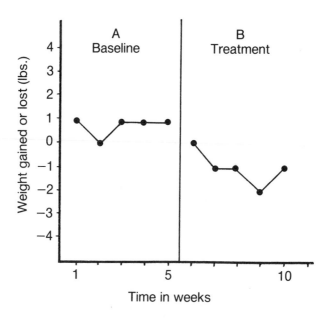

Figure 7.2. Simple line graph indicating the number of pounds gained or lost per week.

Cumulative Graphs

Cumulative graphs are used less frequently in presenting and analyzing data from single system designs. They, nevertheless, represent a graphing strategy that may be appropriate for selected cases. Cumulative graphs are constructed the same as simple line (noncumulative) graphs, except for one important difference. Cumulative graphs differ from simple line graphs in that the amount of behavior recorded for the first session or trial is added or subtracted to the amount of behavior recorded for the second session. The sum of the first two sessions or trials is then added or subtracted to the amount of behavior or performance in the third session, and so on. Continuing with the previous example, Figure 7.3 depicts a cumulative graph of the same data presented in Figure 7.2. In the cumulative graph, the amount of weight gained or lost in 1 week is added or subtracted to the recorded weight in the subsequent weeks. Thus, a cumulative record of the client's total weight loss rather than a record of his week-by-week weight loss is available.

Bar Graph

A simple bar graph or histogram is comprised of a series of columns running vertically or horizontally. The columns represent client per-

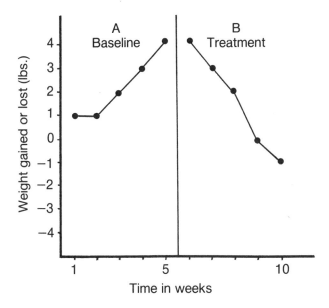

Figure 7.3. Cumulative graph indicating the number of pounds gained or lost over evaluation period.

formance. Bar graphs are traditionally used with discrete data and comparative information. Histograms (bar graphs), however, can be employed with continuous data, in which case each bar often represents the mean or average performance for a separate phase. Figure 7.4 represents such an application of a bar graph to an ABAB design. In this case, each column represents the mean or average performance for that phase for the outcome measure.

A more common use of the bar graph is to present performance across trials or time; multiple bars are used to depict the magnitude of client performance. Figure 7.5 displays the data presented earlier for the simple line graph and the cumulative line graph (the weight reduction example). In this application of the histogram to these data, the client's total weight was used and appears on the y-axis. One bar represents each recording of weight during the baseline and intervention phases.

Bar graphs provide one of the most comprehensible methods of displaying the magnitude of behavior change. Histograms are straightforward and provide an easy-to-construct method of displaying comparisons. Histograms, however, are not the most effective way to present some data. When bar graphs are used to present continuous data or when bars are computed to reflect mean levels of performance, valuable information may be lost. For example, Figure 7.6 presents the same data for a simple line graph and for a bar graph. The columns in the bar graph represent the mean

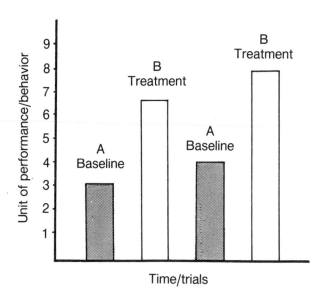

Figure 7.4. Bar graph displaying the average response levels for baseline and treatment periods.

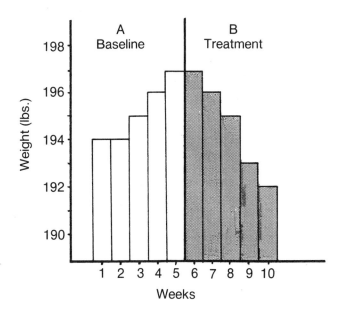

Figure 7.5. Bar graph showing changes in weight per week over baseline and treatment phases.

level of performance for each phase and suggest that there was no difference in performance across the two phases. The simple line graph, however, clearly indicates different response patterns across the two phases. In the baseline phase, client responses were increasing, while in the intervention phase the performance was clearly decreasing. Bar graphs can also obscure variability in data when the columns represent mean or average performance across phases. Figure 7.7 clearly depicts a situation in which variability in response patterns is masked by the presentation of client performance in a bar graph.

Clearly, information presented in bar graphs can be misleading if the therapist is not aware of the limitations of this particular form of graphic analysis. Histograms are useful when data are not continuous within each phase. If continuous data within a phase are presented in a bar graph and mean values are used to represent the columns, the characteristics of the client's response pattern may not be accurately conveyed. In these cases, bar graphs may lead to spurious conclusions based ön visual inspection.

Many types of graphic presentation other than the simple line graph, cumulative line graphs, and bar graphs are possible. These include such alternatives as subdivided line and bar graphs, surface charts, step charts, range graphs, multiple-scale line graphs and deviation graphs, to mention a few. For detailed information on the construction and presentation of these

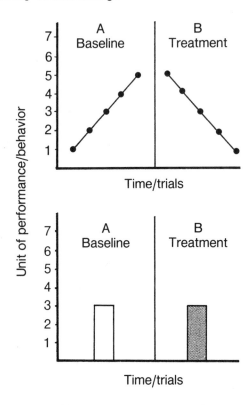

Figure 7.6. Comparison of line graph and bar graph (with the average for each phase used) for the same data series.

more complex and sophisticated methods of graphic analysis, several sources (Parsonson and Baer, 1978; Sander, 1978; Tawney and Gast, 1984) are available.

With the advent of microprocessing technology, computer graphics have the potential to add a new dimension to graphic construction and visual analysis. Three-dimensional charts and graphs can be easily constructed with use of microcomputers. Charts such as the one presented in Figure 7.8 are not widely used presently, but offer an economy of space and provide an interesting and visually appealing format for emphasizing client change across phases and conditions.

General Considerations in Graphic Analysis

The old adage that one picture is worth a thousand words is literally true in relation to the construction and presentation of graphs. In order for graphic methods to convey information accurately, the graphs must be

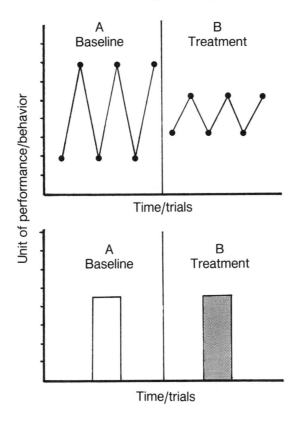

Figure 7.7. Comparison of line graph and bar graph (with the average for each phase used) for the same data.

properly constructed. Because visual impressions are susceptible to influence from distortions, it is important to check the construction of graphs thoroughly before the data they contain are analyzed and judged.

One area in which distortion may be introduced is in the scaling of the x-axis and y-axis. Distortions of scaling are much more commonly associated with the vertical axis or y-axis (representing units of behavior or performance) than with the horizontal axis or x-axis (representing time or trials). For most performance data, vertical changes usually express change related to intervention, and often these changes are the ones that the presentor wishes to emphasize. Figure 7.9 displays two graphs of identical sets of data with different scaling on the y-axis. Figure 7.9, *graph A,* suggests that a trend or change in response pattern occurred across the two phases, while the data in Figure 7.9, *graph B,* present a much less convincing display of a treatment effect.

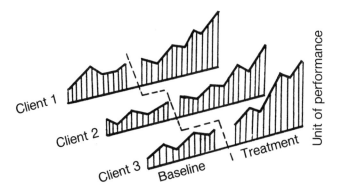

Figure 7.8. Schematic of computer-generated graph for a multiple baseline design across subjects.

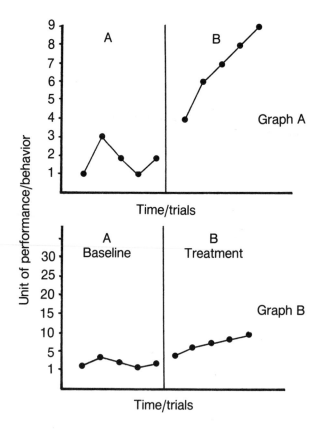

Figure 7.9. Line graphs comparing the same data series, with different scaling used on the y-axis.

To help avoid misinterpretations of graphed data, authorities generally recommend that the scaling units for the y-axis and x-axis be equal or that a 2:3 ratio be used (Kazdin, 1982; Parsonson and Baer, 1978). Tawney and Gast (1984, p. 153) state that the 2:3 y-axis to x-axis ratio "is viewed by researchers as limiting the degree or perceptual distortion. If the ordinate scale (y-axis) were longer than this recommended proportion, a steeper slope in the data path would be present, exaggerating the magnitude of change." A longer space between data points on the x-axis than that allowed by the 2:3 ratio distorts the data visually by conveying a shallow data path (see Figure 7.9B).

Some authorities employ logarithmic scaling conventions in the graphs they use. An example of a semilogarithmic scale in which the y-axis was logarithmic and the x-axis was equal interval scaling is presented in Chapter 4 (see Figure 4.1). This graphic recording form is referred to as the Standard Behavior Chart (White and Haring, 1980). When a semilogarithmic format such as the Standard Behavior Chart is used, the numbers along both scales are arithmetic, but the y-axis is not equal interval and has no zero origin.

The advocates of the Standard Behavior Chart and other ratio charts (White and Haring, 1980; Koorland and Martin, 1975) argue that the semilogarithmic format is ideal for expressing relative comparative rates of change in performance. Despite the wide range of data that can be plotted on the chart and the advantages of the semilogarithmic format, it has not been widely adopted in applied settings. Parsonson and Baer (1978) note that a frequent objection to the use of semilogarithmic scales is that they are often used inappropriately or misinterpreted. A therapist who wishes to use the semilogarithmic convention to graph data should have a good understanding of the difference between semilogarithmic and nonlogarithmic methods of grahic analysis. Several sources (Koorland and Martin, 1975; Pennypacker et al., 1972; White and Haring, 1980) provide the practitioner with this information.

In addition to scaling procedures, there are several other rules that should be followed in presenting data graphically. The phases or experimental conditions should be clearly delineated. This is conventionally done by using a bold solid vertical line between phase changes. Modifications of an intervention within a phase may be indicated by using thinner dashed vertical lines. All vertical lines used to separate treatment conditions should be drawn between the data points.

As noted previously, data points within a phase and across phases are often connected by lines. These lines are then referred to as data paths. Frequently, a graph may contain more than one data path. The use of multiple data paths may be confusing, and the general recommendation is to include no more than three separate data paths within one graph. If more than one data path is included in a graph, the data points associated with each data path may be distinctly marked with use of geometric forms such as circles, triangles, and squares, or the data paths themselves may be represented by different forms of data lines.

Finally, the graph should be labeled clearly and logically. The unit of behavior and/or performance should be concisely and accurately labeled on the y-axis, and the frequency with which data was collected should be labeled on the x-axis. Legends indicating the purpose of the graph should be concise and explanatory. The various phases should be clearly labeled to allow easy identification of the design, and the scaling system should be simple and easy to read. Fractions or decimals should be avoided in the labeling of the intervals along the x-axis and y-axis.

_____ PATTERNS IN VISUAL INSPECTION _____

Assuming that the appropriate graphic methods have been employed, the therapist begins visual inspection which involves the ability to interpret data presented in a graphic format and to derive the appropriate clinical implications. Several components or properties of graphically presented data have been identified as meaningful in the visual inspection of single system data (Wolery and Harris, 1982). The major variations in graphic analysis for which a therapist should be looking are changes in level, variability, trend, and slope.

Visual Components of Graphs

Level. Level refers to what Bloom and Fischer (1982) call changes in the "magnitude" of the data. Changes in level represent changes in the value of a data series as measured on the outcome variable at the point of intervention. In other words, a change in level refers to the shift or discontinuity of client performance from the end of one phase to the beginning of the next phase. Figure 7.10 presents an example of a change in level across phases.

It is noteworthy that a change in level represents an abrupt rise or fall in performance that occurs immediately after the intervention is introduced or withdrawn.

Changes in the magnitude of the data may be conveyed by a change in mean level. A change in mean level across phases or conditions refers to a modification in the average rate of performance across two or more phases. The mean level of performance is computed by adding all the values on the y-axis for a phase and dividing that sum by the sum of the data points. The mean line is then drawn parallel to the abscissa at that value. In Figure 7.10, the mean value for the data in the baseline phase is 2.3 (3 + 1 + 2 + 3 + 2 +

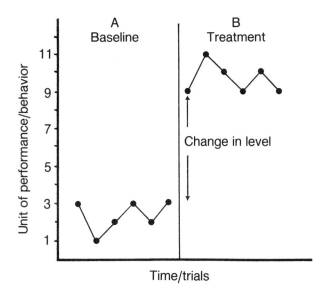

Figure 7.10.   Line graph illustrating change in level from baseline to intervention.

3 = 14/6 = 2.3), and the mean value for the intervention phase is 9.7 (9 +11 + 10 + 9 + 10 + 9 = 58/6 = 9.7). Figure 7.11 illustrates the mean lines for the raw data previously presented in Figure 7.10. In this example, the mean lines clearly indicate that a change in mean level has occurred.

The use of mean lines to emphasize visually changes in mean level of performance can be misleading. For example, if there is an upward or a downward trend in the data or if there is steady predictable improvement in client performance, mean lines may erroneously suggest a clear but spurious change in performance due to intervention. Figure 7.12 presents such an example.

Visual inspection of the raw data in Figure 7.12 clearly reveals that there is a steady improvement in client performance and that the introduction of treatment had no visible effect on a naturally occurring response pattern. The mean lines are also presented and falsely suggest that a change in mean level occurred with the introduction of the intervention. Obviously, this change in level is an artifact of the use of mean values and distorts the actual data pattern.

Mean lines may also be misinterpreted if there is a reversal in the direction of the response patterns across phases. For example, Figure 7.13 indicates a change in the direction of the client's performance across phases. Calculation of mean levels of performance across the phases masks this change in performance and erroneously suggests that the intervention had no effect on the client's performance.

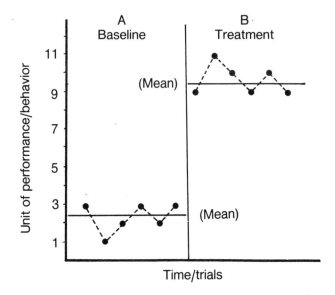

Figure 7.11. Line graph showing mean level of performance for each phase.

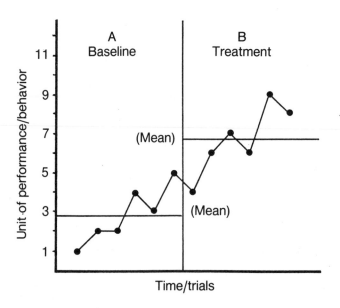

Figure 7.12. Line graph and mean level of performance for baseline and treatment phases.

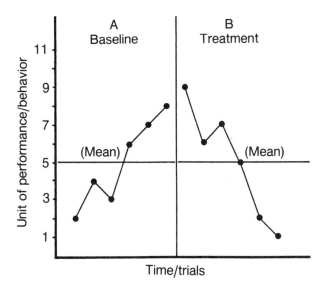

Figure 7.13.   Line graph and mean level of performance for baseline and treatment phases.

When mean levels of data are computed, the mean lines should be displayed over the graph of the raw data to reduce the chance of misinterpretation. Mean levels of performance do not actually "misrepresent" data, although they may be easily misinterpreted. Cautions, therefore, should be directed not to the plotting of mean values per se but to the interpretations that may be made from those values.

Finally, it is important to remember that changes in level refer to the difference or "discontinuity in performance" from the last day or trial in one phase to the first day or trial in the next phase. The therapist is interested in whether the shift in performance that coincides with the introduction of intervention is greater than that which would be expected from ordinary fluctuations or variability in performance.

Variability. Variability refers to the amount of fluctuation or the spread of data points in a series. Excessive variability in the data indicates that the data are unstable and may prevent any meaningful conclusions from being drawn regarding the effectiveness of intervention. This is particularly true if a stable response pattern cannot be obtained during the baseline phase. The amount of variability that can be tolerated in a data series is not agreed upon by authorities in fields such as clinical psychology in which single system procedures are widely used. Some experts have developed guidelines to quantify variability. Tawney and Gast (1984) suggest that 80% to 90% of the data points in a series or phase should fall within a 15% range of the mean level for that phase. If this criterion is met, they contend, most authorities will consider the data stable. This set of guidelines is not universally accepted, however (Bloom and Fischer, 1982).

The method recommended by Tawney and Gast (1984) provides a numerical estimate of the physical variability in a series of data. Limiting the concept of variability to that of a physical property or characteristic of the data has some distinct disadvantages. Barlow et al. (1984) argue that estimates of variability only have meaning within the context with which the data will be interpreted. They contend that variability is a relative concept and should be interpreted in a relative manner. The amount or degree of variability that can be tolerated within a given phase or condition depends on a variety of factors. It depends on knowledge of the treatment procedures and their effects; on knowledge of the behavior, disorder or deficiency and its known course or its response to treatment; on knowledge of the measurement and recording system and how sensitive it is to actual changes in performance; and on knowledge of the effects of a whole series of external conditions and extraneous variables that impact on any attempt to evaluate the effects of an intervention with a specific client in a particular setting. Therapists are often in the best position to judge how much variability is tolerable. One crucial factor is the degree of change that is anticipated due to the intervention. A greater degree of variability can be tolerated if the clinician expects a sudden and substantial treatment effect than if the clinician expects treatment effects to be gradual.

If the intervention is likely to influence the degree of variability of the data, a greater degree of variability in the preceding phase can be accepted. Indeed, in some cases, the degree of variability in a client's response pattern may be the target dimension (see Figure 7.14).

Variability, if it is believed to be excessive, may be reduced by identifying specific environmental factors that appear to be causing fluctuations and by removing them. Parsonson and Baer (1978) note that a systematic search of environmental variables thought to affect variability may lead to the identification of potentially useful treatment factors. If variables that are associated with peaks in the client's response pattern can be identified, these factors may be investigated as potentially powerful treatment components. If variables or environmental factors are associated with dramatic decreases in performance in the data series, these variables may be potential confounds, and their elimination or control may increase the effectiveness of the intervention.

A more formal statistical method does exist for evaluating the effect of variability. The procedure referred to as the C-statistic can provide a numeric estimate of stability. Essentially, the C-statistic compares the overall variability in the data set to the variability which occurs from one data point to the next (Tryon, 1982). This comparison allows the therapist

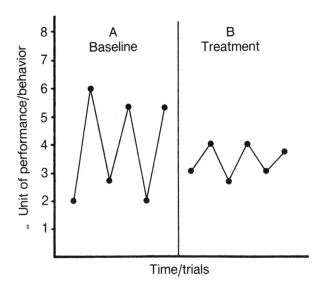

Figure 7.14. Line graph illustrating change in variability across baseline and intervention phases.

to make quantitative statements about variability and about the presence or absence of trends in the data. The C-statistic can also be used to evaluate changes in client performance across phases and is presented in more detail in Chapter 8.

In some cases, none of these methods will be suitable to reduce the variability in a particular evaluation. In such a situation, the lower the amount of physical variation in the data series, the better. The clinical therapist may not have the time or resources to adjust the situation until an extremely stable response pattern is produced. In such a case, the experienced therapist should strive simply to implement the best possible assessment. Applied evaluation with use of systematic methods will always be preferable to no evaluation of client performance, regardless of the limitations of that evaluation attempt.

Trend. Trend refers to the direction in which a response pattern or series of data points is progressing. A response pattern that is systematically increasing may be describing an accelerating trend, while a data series that is consistently decreasing may suggest a decelerating trend. A trend may also be curvilinear or quadratic. Figure 7.15 illustrates three separate data patterns corresponding to an accelerating trend (*A*), a decelerating trend (*B*), and a quadratic trend (*C*).

Changes in trend are reflected by a change in the direction in which the data pattern is moving. Generally, changes in trend are associated with the

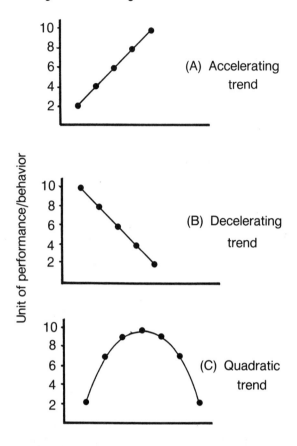

Figure 7.15. Line graphs depicting common data patterns. *Graph A* illustrates an accelerating trend; *graph B,* a decelerating trend; and *graph C,* a quadratic or curvilinear trend.

introduction of the intervention. A change in direction of a client's response pattern is suggestive of a change in performance related to treatment. Figure 7.16 depicts a typical response pattern in which a change in trend occurs across the phases. In the baseline phase, there is a slightly decelerating trend. Following the introduction of treatment, there is a definite change in direction of the response pattern, and an accelerating trend is obvious. In the final phase of the design, when the treatment is withdrawn, there again is a change in direction of the data series; this change is associated with a decelerating trend.

Sometimes variability in the data series makes the detection of a trend difficult. Under such circumstances, several trend plotting procedures are available to assist in the visual analysis of trend within or across phases of

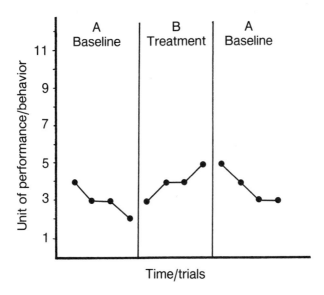

Figure 7.16.   Line graph illustrating the change in trend across phases. In phase A, there is a decelerating trend; in phase B, an accelerating trend; and in the second A phase, a decelerating trend.

the design. These procedures include the freehand method, several semi-average methods, and the method of least squares. The freehand method (Edwards, 1967) consists of drawing a straight line (freehand) that bisects the data points into two equal halves. Without considerable experience and skill, the reliability of judgments of "best fit" with use of the freehand method of trend estimation are likely to be low (Tawney and Gast, 1984). The method of least squares is a more accurate and sophisticated procedure for developing trend lines. Its primary advantage is that it can be used to establish logarithmic, quadratic, or straight line trends in a data series (Dubois, 1964). Its primary disadvantage is that it involves relatively complex statistical computation and thus is not likely to be routinely employed by therapists in clinical settings.

A number of "semiaveraging" procedures are available to assist the clinician in computing trend lines. These trend lines may serve as a valuable adjunct to visual inspection. The most popular is the procedure developed by White (1974), presented by White and Haring (1980), and called the "split-middle" procedure or the celeration line approach.

The objective of the celeration line approach is to fit a trend line to the data points within a phase such that the line approximates a "best fit" of the observed trend in the data. In most cases, the trend line will divide the data points in half so that about half the observations will fall above or on the trend line and half will fall on or below the line. This line is often referred to as a celeration line, which suggests that the response pattern in that phase may be accelerating, decelerating, or stationary.

Generally, the celeration line is computed for the baseline phase and then extended into the intervention phase. The purpose of extending the celeration line into the intervention phase is to predict the trend of the client's responses. If the treatment procedure has no effect on the client's response pattern during the intervention phase, the same proportion of data points will fall above and below the celeration line during the intervention phase as fell during the baseline phase. If, on the other hand, there is a change in the client's response pattern during the intervention phase, the proportion of data points above or below the celeration line will change during the treatment phase. The above description assumes that there is a *linear* trend for the data points in each phase.

An example will help illustrate how the celeration line approach may be utilized. The following steps are completed to compute the celeration line.

Step 1. In order to determine whether there has been any change in the client's response pattern related to intervention, it is necessary to measure client performance over two or more phases. In the simplest example, the first period of measurement consists of the pretreatment baseline period. The client's performance during the intervention phase is then compared to that observed during the baseline period. A set of baseline data for a hypothetical client appear in Figure 7.17, *graph A*.

Baseline data are collected and plotted on a graph, as described previously. The client's behavior or performance is recorded on the vertical axis (y-axis) and the time or trials on the horizontal axis (x-axis). White (1977) recommends that a minimum of eight to ten observations or data points be recorded in the baseline for the use of the celeration line approach. Fewer than ten data points may be used, but this is likely to result in a less accurate fitting celeration line for the baseline performance (Kazdin, 1976).

Step 2. The baseline data are divided in half by drawing a solid vertical line separating the first half of the sessions from the second half (see Figure 7.17, *graph B*). When the baseline phase includes an odd number of data points, the vertical line should be drawn through the middle data point. Next, divide each of the halves in half by drawing dashed vertical lines (see Figure 7.17, *graph C*). Again, if there is an odd number of data points during each half of the baseline phase, draw the dashed line through the middle data point.

Step 3. The median level of performance is determined for each half of the baseline data. The median is the score that divides the data equally in

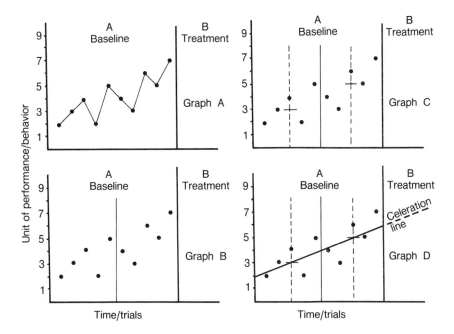

Figure 7.17.   Line graphs depicting the steps involved in computing the celeration line. *Graph A* is the original data series. In *graph B*, the baseline data series is divided in half. In *graph C*, each half of the baseline is divided in half again (*dashed vertical lines*), and the median values are marked on the *dashed lines*. In *graph D*, the celeration line is drawn. (See text for complete explanation).

half. This median is computed from y-axis data points that represent the client's performance. To determine the data point that is the median within each half phase, merely count from the bottom up on the y-axis toward the top data point for each half phase of the baseline. Once this data point is determined, a horizontal line is drawn through it at each half phase until the line intersects the dashed vertical line made earlier. For example, in Figure 7.17, *graph B*, there are five data points in the first half phase of the baseline. They are 2, 2, 3, 4, 5, as measured on the y-axis labeled Unit of Performance/Behavior. The median for this group of scores is 3. Therefore, a horizontal line is drawn that intersects the first dashed vertical line at the level of 3 on the y-axis (see Figure 7.17, *graph C*). For the second half of the baseline the response values are 3, 4, 5, 6, 7, as indicated on the y-axis. The median for this group of scores is 5, and a horizontal line intersecting the second dashed vertical line is drawn at the level of 5 on the y-axis (see Figure 7.17, *graph C*).

Although most authors (Kazdin, 1982; Tawney and Gast, 1984; White and Haring, 1980; Wolery and Harris, 1982) recommend use of the median value of the scores in each half phase of the baseline, some authorities (Bloom and Fischer, 1982) suggest computing the mean value instead of the median for the data points in each half phase.

Step 4. The next step is to draw a straight line through the two intersections of the dashed lines created in the previous step. This line is referred to as the celeration line (see Figure 7.17, *graph D*).

Step 5. The celeration line should be adjusted up or down so that it comes as close as possible to dividing the baseline data into two equal halves. In Figure 7.17, *graph D*, there is no need to make this adjustment, since the line already equally divides the data points. This may not always occur naturally, and in some cases the line may have to be raised or lowered slightly to achieve this effect. The adjusted line must remain parallel to the original line.

Step 6. The final step is to extend the celeration or trend line calculated in the baseline phase into the intervention phase. Then the data series during treatment is compared to that predicted by the response pattern observed during the baseline phase. Figure 7.18 presents the use of a celeration line to compare response patterns of a child with learning disabilities (Ot-

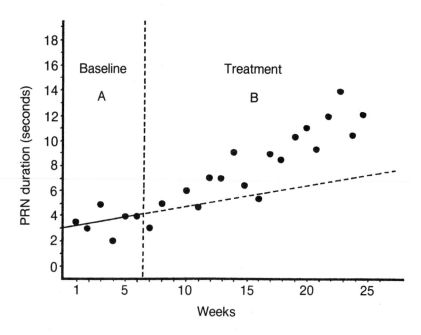

Figure 7.18. Demonstration of celeration line procedure on a clinically obtained data series. *PRN,* postrotary nystagmus. (Adapted from: Ottenbacher, K. (1983). Patterns of postrotary nystagmus in three learning disabled children. *Am. J. Occup. Ther., 36,* 657–663.)

tenbacher, 1983). In this case, the outcome variable measured during a baseline and an intervention period was the child's duration of postrotary nystagmus. The response pattern for the treatment phase is substantially different from that for the baseline phase.

The celeration line, or any trend line, is only an estimate of trend designed to facilitate visual inspection and, like the mean level, can divert attention away from the point-by-point data path.

Slope. The final component of visual inspection is slope. Slope refers to the change in pitch or angle of a trend; in other words, it refers to the steepness of a data path (trend line) across time. Figure 7.19 illustrates a change in slope across the two phases but no change in direction or trend.

The slope of a trend line can be expressed numerically by dividing two points along the line. For example, in Figure 7.20 the slope of the celeration line can be computed by taking the value of the celeration line at one point along the x-axis and dividing it by another. The x-axis in Figure 7.20 is divided into days. A common procedure is to compute the slope of the trend line as an indication of rate of change or progress over time. Generally, the rate of change is computed over a week-long period. This procedure can easily be applied to Figure 7.20. At day 1 on the x-axis, the celeration line is at 10. Seven days later, the line is at approximately 15. The slope of the line

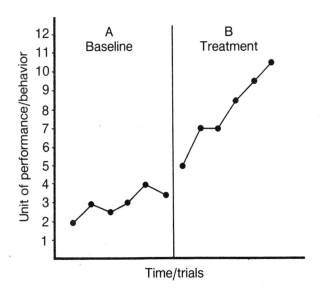

Figure 7.19. Line graph showing data series that demonstrates change in slope across baseline and treatment phases.

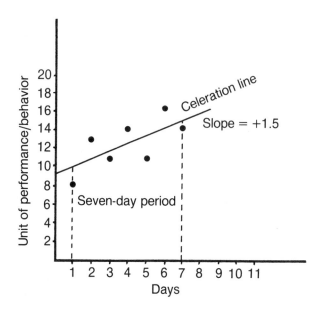

Figure 7.20.   Celeration line and slope for 7-day data series.

is computed by dividing 15 by 10 (15/10) which results in a slope of 1.5. The 1.5 is labeled as positive, since it is moving in an upward direction. Because the line is accelerating, this suggests that the average rate of responding during the week for which the slope was computed is ∓1.5 times greater than it was during the prior week. This ratio expressing the slope of the celeration line provides a convenient and easy-to-calculate method for providing a numeric index of rate of client change over time. The slopes of trend lines for separate baseline and intervention phases may be computed and compared to provide the therapist with a quantitative indication of rate of change from baseline to intervention phase.

Common Patterns

The visual components of graphs, including level, variability, trend, and slope, constitute the foundation which graphic analysis and visual inspection of single system data are based. Visual inspection is conducted by judging the extent to which changes in these components are evident across phases and whether the changes are consistent with the requirements of the particular design. Figure 7.21 depicts a number of common data patterns in which the mean line is used to depict performance across phases. In Figure 7.21, *A* illustrates a change in level across phases but no change in trend or slope, *B* and *C* depict changes in trend (direction) but no change in level, *D*

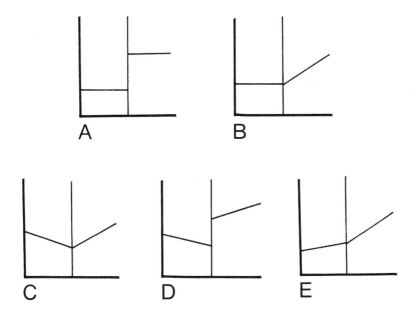

Figure 7.21.   Line graphs illustrating common response patterns. *Graph A* shows a change in level, *graphs B* and *C* show changes in trend (direction), *graph D* shows both a change in trend and a change in level, and *graph E* depicts a change in slope but no change in trend or level.

illustrates both a change in trend and a change in level, and *E* illustrates a change in slope but no change in trend or level. There is no change in trend in Figure 7.21*E* because the direction of the data across the phases has not changed (it continues to accelerate). Only the angle or slope of the line is different from one phase to the next.

Clearly, the data patterns presented in Figure 7.21 are illustrative only. Hundreds of possible data patterns may occur. These potential data configurations will be affected by multiple factors or background characteristics that may influence visual inspection. Whether a particular data pattern will be considered indicative of a clinically significant treatment effect will depend on the variability of performance within a particular phase, the length of the phase, the number of data points collected, the consistency of the pattern across phases, the reliability of the measurement procedures, and other related factors. In practice, changes in level, variability, trend, and slope occur simultaneously, which makes visual inspection of data an art that requires considerable practice and expertise. Often, patterns of data that appear to be indicating only one visual characteristic may, on closer inspection and analysis, be found to exhibit several characteristics.

As noted in Chapter 5, in the typical ABAB design it is commonly expected that a reversal to baseline levels should occur during the second phase and that this is a common visual characteristic that therapists examining an ABAB design may be looking for in graphic analysis. As also suggested in Chapter 5, however, a reversal of client performance to baseline is not a requirement of the design. Hayes (1981) notes that a pattern of data such as that presented in Figure 7.22A is indicative of a strong treatment effect despite the fact that there is only a leveling off of client performance during the second A phase and not a complete reversal. The argument is made that if visual inspection indicates that performance improves faster during the treatment phase than during the baseline and withdrawal phases, there is evidence for a treatment effect. Visually, it may be instructive to regraph the data presented in Figure 7.22A to underscore this fact.

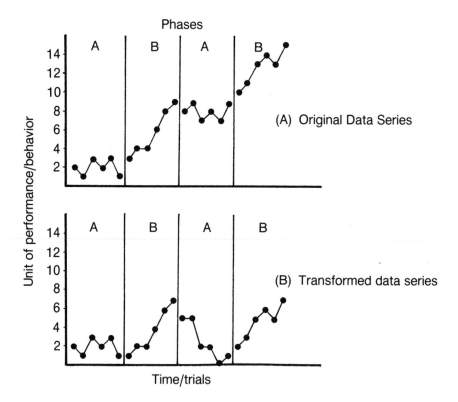

Figure 7.22. Line graphs illustrating response patterns for ABAB design. The second A phase in the original data series (*graph A*) does not evidence a reversal to baseline level. In *graph B*, the original data series has been regraphed as difference scores from the trend in the previous phase.

The data in Figure 7.22*A* represent a typical ABAB design in which withdrawal produces less improvement in the second A phase but no reversal to baseline levels. In the second B phase, intervention when reintroduced continues to be associated with a treatment effect; i.e., an accelerating trend. In Figure 7.22*B*, the data have been regraphed to demonstrate visually the effect of the intervention. Figure 7.22*B* shows the same data plotted as difference scores from the trend in the previous phase. In this procedure, a trend line is computed for a phase, and the data points from the next phase are sequentially subtracted from the corresponding data point on the trend line. For example, the first data point in the first B phase is subtracted from the trend value of 2 which was computed for the first A phase. In the A phase the trend is a horizontal line, and therefore all the values in the first B phase will be subtracted from the same number (i.e., 2). When the trend line is computed for the first B phase, it will be accelerating, and the values will be different for each corresponding value of the second A phase. This procedure results in a graph in which data are plotted in terms of improvement relative to trends recorded in previous phases. With use of this simple procedure, the classic reversal pattern emerges from the data presented previously in Figure 7.22*A*. What is reversing in this case is not the level of behavior, but the trends across phases. Both procedures are accurate but present different visual images to evaluate. This example clearly illustrates that the art of visual inspection requires considerable expertise and skill and is not as simple or as easy as might initially be assumed. Visual inspection involves more than simply "eyeballing" the plotted data and arbitrarily deciding whether the data reflect a treatment effect. Several characteristics of the data must be examined and evaluated. The descriptive aids presented in previous sections of this chapter can facilitate graphic examination and enhance the visual interpretation of data.

ADVANTAGES OF GRAPHIC ANALYSIS AND VISUAL INSPECTION

Graphic analysis and visual inspection are accepted methods of data reduction in much applied behavior research. These procedures have a number of advantages for evaluating change in clinical or therapeutic settings. The techniques are applicable with only a single client or a small group of clients. In contrast, many of the formal data analysis procedures used in the behavioral and social sciences require multiple participants and, therefore, are not practical for use in many evaluations of clinical outcome in which the number of clients receiving the treatment is very small.

Visual analysis is also a dynamic process. The data are recorded and plotted on a continuous basis. The graph allows the therapist to systematically include all the client's responses over a period of time. Thus, visual analysis of data patterns encourages the investigation of process as well as outcome. The convention of continuous recording and graphing of client performance also increases the chance of detecting findings of therapeutic relevance which may not be directly related to the problem under treatment but may have important implications for future intervention.

Visual analysis provides the therapist with an accepted empirical method of judging whether the treatment effect is clinically significant. As noted previously, visual analysis of the data should reveal only those intervention effects that are powerful enough to have produced clinically meaningful results. The insensitivity of visual analysis to "weak" treatment effects that are not obvious by simply looking at the graphed data is considered a major advantage of visual inspection by some authorities. Parsonson and Baer (1978) argue that the potency of treatment effects revealed through visual inspection assures the therapist that the intervention effects are important and reliable because they appear despite use of a relatively insensitive measurement process. They (1978, p. 114) go on to argue that intervention effects demonstrated through visual analysis are likely to be "basic" and associated with "a widespread sphere of influence with respect to the phenomenon of interest. Thus, basic variables have powerful and generalizable effects, and their discovery provides the impetus for the development of an area of scientific inquiry."

Finally, graphic presentation is relatively easy to develop and is widely understood and comprehended by a variety of professional and non-professional persons who will have an interest in the client's performance during treatment. Graphic analysis allows the interested party to evaluate the range and stability of client performance and the degree of control obtained and to determine whether the requirements of a particular design were met.

Because of these characteristics, graphic analysis and visual inspection have been accepted as practical and useful methods for evaluating client performance and are widely employed by clinicians, educators, and professionals evaluating individual client change.

DISADVANTAGES OF GRAPHIC ANALYSIS AND VISUAL INSPECTION

One of the major criticisms of graphic analysis and visual inspection of single system data has been the lack of any formal decision rules or guidelines associated with visual inspection, i.e., no theoretical framework to guide visual interpretation. As a result, the process of visual inspection and visual inference has received very little empirical attention. No theoretical framework is available that can be used to examine the process of visual inference and to empirically test hypotheses generated from a theoretical perspective (Furlong and Wampold, 1981, 1982; Wampold and Furlong, 1981). As Kazdin (1982, p. 239) has noted, "perhaps the major issue pertains to the lack of concrete decision rules for determining whether a particular demonstration shows or fails to show a reliable effect. The process of visual inspection would seem to permit, if not actively encourage, subjectivity and inconsistency in the evaluation of intervention effects."

Research investigating the reliability of visual inspection across different examiners has revealed a cause for concern. Jones et al. (1978) compared judges' use of visual inference with time-series analysis of single system data and found that there was often poor agreement between visual and statistical methods of data analysis and that interjudge agreement for visual analysis was low. In a similar study, DeProspero and Cohen (1979) developed hypothetical graphs and then had experienced reviewers of behaviorally oriented psychology journals rate the degree of "experimental control" shown in the graphic data. They found that interjudge agreement was low. Gottman and Glass (1978), White (1971), and Wampold and Furlong (1981) have also provided evidence that visual inspection may result in inconsistent and unreliable interpretations of a data series in some cases. Many of these authorities have advocated the use of some form of statistical analysis in conjunction with visual inspection of single system data. The role of statistical procedures in the analysis of single system data is discussed in Chapter 8.

Another limitation of visual inspection is that it considers only those effects that in the plotted data can easily be seen as significant. This relates back to the issue of clinical significance versus statistical significance which was discussed earlier. The problem with overemphasizing the importance of "clinical" significance is that consistent but relatively "weak" treatment effects may be overlooked by reliance on visual inspection. Kazdin (1982) points out that when a treatment program is first being developed and tested, it may produce only "weak" treatment effects that may be overlooked by visual inspection. If the treatment approach were developed and refined, it might eventually be capable of producing powerful treatment effects. By reliance on only visual inspection during the initial stage of evaluating an intervention procedure, it is possible that some potentially useful treatment methods could be abandoned prematurely because they did not produce a large treatment effect easily detected by visual inspection. This would be comparable to making a Type II experimental error in group-comparison research, in which a null hypothesis is falsely supported when it should have been rejected.

A final problem with visual inspection of a data series collected from a single client is that the data may be distorted or misinterpreted due to the presence of serial dependency within the data. Data collected in single system designs is invariably of a repeated nature. That is, measurements on the outcome variable are taken repeatedly of the performance of an individual or small group over time. That repeated measurements are gathered from a client means that there is a degree of serial dependency or autocorrelation within the data collected. Serial dependency refers to the fact that sequential responses emitted by the same individual will be correlated. The higher the correlation between responses, the better one can predict performance over time. The result of this serial dependency is to reduce the variability in the observed responses and thereby bias "the estimates of behavioral score properties like stabilities, variabilities, or averages" (Jones et al., 1977, p. 155). The presence of serial dependency within a data series adds to the interpretive difficulties based solely on visual inspection. Observed changes may actually have been quite predictable because of the serial dependency. An apparently clear visual pattern may be influenced by autocorrelation which may lead to a misinterpretation of the findings if only graphic analysis and visual inspection are used to evaluate the data (see Gottman and Glass, 1978; and Jones et al., 1978). Cook and Campbell (1979) present a detailed discussion of the problems caused by serial dependency and describe several quantitative procedures designed to deal with the effect of autocorrelation in a data series. Autocorrelation and its effect on data from single system designs is discussed in more detail in Chapter 8.

CONCLUSIONS

Graphic analysis and visual inspection are valuable data-analytic tools in evaluating response patterns associated with single system designs. Graphs present visual summaries of data and provide information to the therapist concerning possible functional relationships between intervention procedures and client performance. In addition, graphic analysis provides a record of client performance over time and presents the data in such a manner that it is easily understood and assimilated by clients and therapists alike.

Graphic analysis and visual inspection are efficient and economical ways to evaluate data. Graphs communicate information related to changes in level, variability, trend, and slope in client response data. Accurate analysis of the various components associated with visual analysis will enhance a therapist's ability to make decisions regarding client treatment.

Parsonson and Baer (1978) contend that there are four factors which help graphs to serve an important evaluative function—clarity, simplicity, explicitness, and good design. The material presented in this chapter should help therapists to understand and incorporate these four factors in the graphic analysis and visual inspection used with their clients.

CHAPTER **8**

Statistical Analysis of Single System Data

INTRODUCTION

Visual analysis or what Sidman (1960) refers to as "criterion by inspection" is the standard method of data evaluation employed by practitioners using single system designs. As noted in Chapter 7, however, relying exclusively on graphic analysis and visual inspection has some serious limitations, and applied researchers and clinicians are beginning to advocate the use of alternative or adjunctive data analysis strategies. For example, Christensen (1980, p. 261) has observed that "as single subject designs have become more popular in the applied research areas, there has been increased emphasis on the need for statistical analysis of the collected data." The use of various statistical techniques with single system designs is controversial. Several authorities (Baer, 1977; Michael, 1974) believe that it is inappropriate to employ statistical techniques with single system designs and argue that the application of statistical procedures confuses the issue of clinical significance with that of statistical significance. Hersen and Barlow (1976) present an excellent overview of the arguments surrounding the issue of clinical significance as they relate to single system designs.

RATIONALE FOR AND AGAINST THE USE OF STATISTICAL PROCEDURES

Kazdin (1982) has outlined several major sources of controversy that are associated with the use of statistical procedures in single system evaluations. The first concern relates to the general appropriateness of statistical procedures in any applied investigation of individual performance. This concern encompasses the issue of clinical versus statistical significance and several other issues introduced in Chapter 7. These include the need to identify only powerful interventions that will produce large treatment effects and have wide generalizability as well as concerns that statistical significance may be misinterpreted and that researchers will rely on statistical procedures to control or manipulate intrasubject variability rather than on improvement of the designs or interventions (Baer, 1977; Michael, 1974).

Despite these acknowledged limitations (Bakan, 1966; Carver, 1978), there is a growing recognition of the possible benefits of statistically analyzing data collected in single system evaluation studies. Kazdin (1982) has identified four situations in which statistical procedures may be warranted. The first of these situations is when the baseline data are unstable. Visual inspection relies heavily on the presence of a stable baseline to serve as a standard for comparison. If the performance during the baseline period is variable or indicates an accelerating or decelerating trend, the performance in subsequent phases may be very difficult to interpret (DeProspero and Cohen, 1979; Furlong and Wampold, 1981). Statistical procedures can be helpful in determining whether a reliable intervention effect has occurred beyond what would have been expected by a continuation of a baseline trend.

The second situation in which statistical procedures may be useful is in the initial stages of investigating a new intervention or treatment. As noted in Chapter 7, visual inspection is dependent on the presence of large or dramatic changes in client performance from one phase to the next. This reliance is functional, in that such changes are likely to be associated with powerful treatments that will produce clinically meaningful results (Parsonson and Baer, 1978). The therapist working with a new treatment program or intervention strategy, however, is probably engaging in some trial-and-error applications of the treatment and is likely to be unfamiliar with conditions and procedures that will maximize the treatment's effectiveness. Initially, the treatment program may produce relatively weak but consistent treatment effects. With time and experience, the therapist may be able to refine the intervention so that its effects on client performance are large and clinically significant. Such interventions should not be abandoned prematurely because they do not immediately produce large treatment effects that are readily apparent on visual inspection. Even if the treatment does not evolve to produce large treatment effects, it may be an important facilitator when it is combined with another related intervention. Statistical analysis can detect small and reliable intervention effects which may then be further developed and refined.

The third situation in which statistical procedures may be a valuable adjunct to visual analysis is when there is a relatively large degree of intrasubject variability in the treatment setting. As single system strategies are adapted and applied in clinical settings, the opportunities for traditional experimental control over variables associated with client performance markedly decreases. As single system methods are applied in field settings, "experimental" control is reduced and the variability of client performance increases. To make judgments based only on visual inspection of the data becomes increasingly difficult with larger intraclient variability in performance. Statistical procedures can enhance the decision-making process when there is considerable variability in client responses.

The final reason for using statistical procedures that has been identified by Kazdin (1982) is that small improvements not detectable by visual analysis may be significant. The usefulness of the intervention for selected areas cannot always be evaluated in terms of the magnitude of performance for a single individual. Small changes in individual performance may be significant, particularly, if those changes are viewed collectively. In such situations, the intervention may not need to produce large treatment effects to be of practical value. Cooper (1981a) presents an excellent example of a situation in which small effects produce a significant cumulative result. The example has to do with energy consumption and conservation. Cooper (1981a) observed that if a driver keeps his tires properly inflated, he or she will improve gas mileage and reduce gasoline consumption. On an individual basis, the effect of this intervention is small. If this effect is applied across a large enough number of individuals, however, the result is a significant reduction in fuel consumption. Similarly, rehabilitation therapy may reduce the duration of hospital stay or the need to return for further hospitalization by a small amount for any given patient. The monetary savings associated with any one client's reduction in hospital care may be small. The savings could be substantial, however, when aggregated over a large number of clients. Thus, small effects, when accrued over several different individuals or over an extended period of time, may be significant. The use of statistical procedures can contribute to the identification and evaluation of these small effects. As Gilbert et al. (1975, p. 157) have accurately noted, "once small effects are found and documented, it may be possible to build improvements upon them. The banking and insurance businesses have built their fortunes on small effects—effects the size of interest rates."

One additional reason to consider the use of statistical procedures is the presence of serial dependency in data from single system designs. In Chapter 7, serial dependency is briefly defined as a common property of repeated observations of a single subject. As noted also, visual interpretation of a data series is more difficult if there is serial dependency (Hartmann et al., 1980). Jones et al. (1978) compared the interpretation based on graphic analysis and visual inspection to that based on a selected statistical technique (time-series analysis). They found that conclusions based on visual analysis were supported in some cases and not supported in other cases and that the statistical procedures sometimes revealed statistically significant changes in trend or level that were not reported as a part of the visual analysis. The most significant discrepancy between visual inspection and statistical analysis occurred in those data series found to have the most serial dependency. Jones et al. (1978) also found that slightly more than 80% of the studies included in the investigation evidenced a significant degree of serial dependency.

A related demonstration of the difficulty that serial dependency can cause the therapist relying solely on visual inspection was reported by Gottman and Glass (1978). They provided 13 judges with two graphs and asked the judges to visually inspect the graphs and determine whether or not there was an intervention effect. The data series in both graphs evidenced a high degree of serial dependency. In the first graph, a time-series statistical analysis revealed that there was a statistically significant intervention effect; only 7 of 13 judges, however, considered the graphed data to indicate a treatment effect. The second graph evidenced no statistically significant treatment effect based on time-series analysis, yet 11 of 13 judges felt that there was a significant intervention effect. The findings of Glass and Gottman (1978) and others (Hartmann et al., 1980; Jones et al., 1977) clearly demonstrate that analysis based on visual inspection can produce results that vary from judge to judge and that conflict with the results from statistical tests. This disagreement appears to be associated with the presence of serial dependency in a data series. The presence of serial dependency would appear to argue strongly for a reliable assessment strategy to be used in conjunction with visual analysis. As Bloom and Fischer (1982, p. 439) state, ''visual inspection of data should be considered a very useful beginning point. But unless the patterns are very clear, with sufficient numbers of observations and with stable baseline data, other methods of analysis should also be employed.'' These methods of analysis, which are considered throughout the rest of this chapter, include a variety of statistical and semistatistical procedures that can be used to supplement visual inspection.

SERIAL DEPENDENCY

Serial dependency, as stated in Chapter 7, refers to the fact that sequential responses emitted by the same individual will be correlated. The higher the correlation between responses, the more accurate the prediction of performance. Thus, knowing the level of performance of a client at a given time allows one to make predictions about subsequent performance. The extent to which there is dependency among successive observations can be assessed by examining autocorrelation (serial correlation) in the data series. Serial dependency is appraised by computing a statistic called an autocorrelation coefficient. The autocorrelation coefficient indicates the extent to which scores at one point in a series are predictive of scores at another point in the same series. For computing autocorrelation, pairs of scores from the data series are formed as follows. The score from time point 1 is paired with the second score, the score from point 2 (second score) is paired with the third score, and so on. When pairs are formed with scores from adjacent time points, the resultant coefficient is called a lag-1 autocorrelation, since there is a 1 point lag or difference between the two scores in each pair. Larger lags can be formed by pairing score 1 with score 3, score 2 with score 4, and so on. Such a comparison strategy would result in a lag-2 autocorrelation. The autocorrelation is interpreted exactly like the conventional correlation, except that the degrees of freedom for determining the significance of the coefficient are reduced by the number of lags.

If the lag-1 autocorrelation for a series of performance measures from an evaluation is statistically significant ($p < .05$), the scores are said to be serially dependent. Often when the lag-1 autocorrelation is significant, the coefficients for larger lags will also be significant, but usually the size of the correlations decreases as the lag increases. This means that the ability to predict one score or response from another lessens as the lag increases (Glass et al., 1975; McDowall et al., 1980).

As noted previously, to make accurate judgments based on visual inspection is much more difficult when the scores being analyzed are not independent of each other than when they are independent of each other. Unfortunately, serial dependency also interferes with the interpretation of some statistical procedures.

Serial dependency is a property of single system data that has not been widely recognized or well understood by researchers and clinicians in the behavioral and social sciences in spite of the profound effect it may have on data analysis and interpretation. A thorough understanding of serial dependency is a prerequisite for accurate interpretation and analysis of a data series regardless of whether visual inspection or statistical procedures are used. Obviously, determining whether there is serial dependency within a data series should be of concern to therapists using single system evaluation procedures. The steps employed in computing a simple lag-1 autocorrelation follow.

Step 1. Assume that with use of a conventional AB design, a series of data points has been collected for a client. The data points are plotted in Figure 8.1. The scores during the baseline phase are 4, 4, 5, 7, 5, 6, 3, 5, 4, and 7. Now compute the mean of the scores. The mean is 50/10 = 5.

Step 2. Next, calculate a difference value for each score. The value is computed by subtracting each score from the mean value.

Score	−	Mean	=	Difference Value
4	−	5	=	−1
4	−	5	=	−1
5	−	5	=	0
7	−	5	=	2
5	−	5	=	0
6	−	5	=	1
3	−	5	=	−2
5	−	5	=	0
4	−	5	=	−1
7	−	5	=	2

Step 3. Next, take each mean difference value found in step 2 and multiply it by the adjacent value. In other words, multiply the first difference (−1) by the second difference (−1), the second difference (−1) by the third difference (0), and so on, until all the values have been used. Then, add the products.

$$
\begin{aligned}
(-1)\,(-1) &= +1 \\
(-1)\,(0) &= 0 \\
(0)\,(+2) &= 0 \\
(+2)\,(0) &= 0 \\
(0)\,(+1) &= 0 \\
(+1)\,(-2) &= -2 \\
(-2)\,(0) &= 0 \\
(0)\,(-1) &= 0 \\
(-1)\,(+2) &= \underline{-2} \\
\text{Sum} &= -3
\end{aligned}
$$

Step 4. Next, square each of the mean difference values obtained in step 2 and add the results: $(-1)^2 + (-1)^2 + (0)^2 + (-2)^2 + (0)^2 + (+1)^2 + (-2)^2 + (0)^2 + (-1)^2 + (+2)^2 = 16$.

Step 5. Then, divide the results obtained in step 3 by the results obtained in step 4. Disregard the sign for the value obtained in step 3. The result is the autocorrelation coefficient r:

$$\text{Autocorrelation } r = 3/16 = .188$$

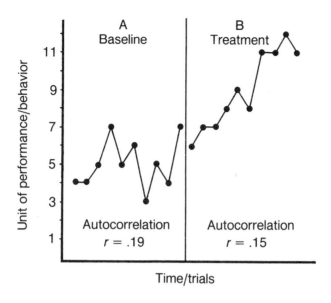

Figure 8.1. Data series for AB design. Autocorrelation coefficients indicating degree of serial dependency have been computed for baseline and treatment phases (see text for procedures used to compute the autocorrelations).

Step 6. For determining whether the autocorrelation coefficient is statistically significant or not, a simple procedure called Bartlett's test may be used. If the autocorrelation coefficient is greater than $2/\sqrt{n}$, where $n =$ the number of baseline observations, the autocorrelation coefficient is considered significant. In the present example, $2/\sqrt{n} = 2/\sqrt{10} = .63$. The obtained autocorrelation coefficient of .188 is not larger than .63. Therefore, the baseline data do not demonstrate a significant degree of autocorrelation.

In Figure 8.1, the autocorrelation coefficient for the data recorded during intervention (B phase) was .15 which was not significant. There is some controversy as to whether the autocorrelation should be computed for just the baseline data, the baseline and intervention data separately, or the entire data series (Gottman and Glass, 1978; Hartmann et al., 1980; Jayaratne and Levy, 1979). Obviously, if the intervention is effective, it could influence the relationship between the data points and contribute a degree of "dependency" that did not exist in the baseline phase. A conservative approach would be to compute autocorrelations for each phase, and if there was a significant coefficient in any phase, the data series should be treated as serially dependent. An exception to this rule would be when there are a very small number of data points in any given phase (e.g., 5 or less). The test used to determine whether the autocorrelation is significant (Bartlett's test) is not sensitive to small *ns*. When there are 5 or fewer data points in a phase, the autocorrelation coefficient should be computed across the entire data series.

A controversy regarding how autocorrelation coefficients should be computed is developing. The procedure described previously is widely accepted and advocated by applied researchers (Jayaratne and Levy, 1979; Jones et al., 1969; Jones et al., 1978). Huitema (1985) recently proposed an alternative method for computing autocorrelation coefficients, with the residuals rather than the raw scores used for a data series. The method proposed by Huitema (1985) generally results in smaller autocorrelation coefficients for a given data set. The resolution of which approach is most appropriate will require additional investigation. Until a consensus is reached among applied scientists and statisticians, the conventional procedure presented previously should continue to serve as the method of computing autocorrelation coefficients.

TRANSFORMATIONS OF AUTOCORRELATED DATA

If the data are not serially dependent, visual inspection along with one of the statistical or semistatistical procedures may be applied directly to the data. A significant autocorrelation coefficient, however, may complicate visual inspection (Jones et al., 1978). The therapist may not be able to confidently apply many statistical procedures if serial dependency is demonstrated. Some statistical tests require that the data points be independent before they can legitimately be applied. Thus, the usefulness of these particular tests and their capability of assisting the therapist in making decisions regarding the effectiveness of treatment are limited. Fortunately, there are a couple of simple methods for removing the serial dependency in a data series. These procedures are easily applied to data collected in clinical settings and include the first difference transformation and the moving average transformation.

First Difference Transformation

The first difference transformation is a simple procedure which is most useful for transforming data that evidences significant autocorrelation and appears to be moving in a linear direction or exhibiting a linear trend. Assume that the data plotted in Figure 8.2 have been collected from a client receiving therapy services. The autocorrelation coefficient was computed, according to the procedures described previously, to be an *r* of .70, which was statistically significant; this means that the data in this series are

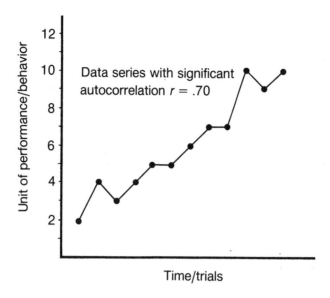

Figure 8.2. Line graph of data series that has a statistically significant degree of autocorrelation.

serially dependent. The following steps are used to perform a first difference transformation of the data.

Step 1. The first score in the data series is subtracted from the second, the second from the third, the third from the fourth, and so on, until all scores are used: $2 - 4 = -2, 4 - 3 = +1, 3 - 4 = -1, 4 - 5 = -1, 5 - 5 = 0, 5 - 6 = -1$, etc. The transformed data are $-2, +1, -1, -1, 0, -1, -1, 0, -3, +1$, and -1. The number of data points has been reduced by one from 12 to 11, since pairs of scores are used with the first difference transformation procedure.

Step 2. With use of the *transformed* data generated in step 1, the autocorrelation is computed to determine whether there is a significant degree of serial dependency left in the data. With use of the procedures described previously, an autocorrelation coefficient of .51 was obtained for the transformed data. This coefficient was examined by use of Bartlett's test and was found to be nonsignificant, which indicates that the first difference transformation had reduced the serial dependency in the data series. The transformed data are presented in Figure 8.3. *Graph A* of Figure 8.3 displays the original data prior to transformation. *Graph B* of Figure 8.3 presents the actual transformed data. This graph contains a number of negative values. In *graph C* of Figure 8.3, a constant of 10 has been added to all the values to remove the minus signs. The data pattern is exactly the

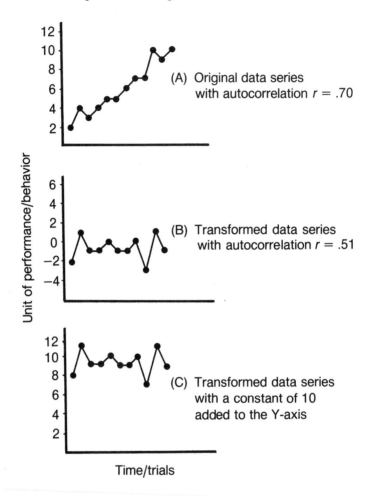

Figure 8.3. Line graphs illustrating original data series (*graph A*), data series transformed with use of the first difference transformation procedure (*graph B*), and the transformed data with a constant of 10 added to remove negative values on the y-axis (*graph C*).

same as that depicted in Figure 8.3, *graph B,* but the values on the ordinate have increased by a constant value to make the graph conform to traditional standards.

If the first difference transformation had not succeeded in removing the serial dependency in the preceding example, an extension of the procedure could have been employed. In this extension, other differentials could be used to achieve the desired transformation. For example, the first score could be subtracted from the third, the second from the fourth, the third from the fifth, and so on. Another option that the therapist can use to eliminate serial dependency from the data series is to employ a moving average transformation.

Moving Average Transformations

As noted previously, first difference transformations are most appropriately used with a data series that evidences a significant autocorrelation coefficient and is displaying a linear trend. If, on the other hand, the data series is associated with a significant autocorrelation and the data appear to be highly variable or evidence much fluctuation, a moving average transformation may be appropriate. The moving average transformation may also be employed when a first difference transformation has failed to reduce the degree of serial dependency in a data series. The moving average transformation is computed in the following manner.

Step 1. Assume that the first difference transformation had not proved a satisfactory method of reducing the autocorrelation in the data presented in Figure 8.2. The therapist may then attempt to "smooth" the data with use of the moving average method. This procedure consists simply of plotting the mean values between two adjacent data points over the entire data series. The paired successive scores and their averages for the data in Figure 8.2 follow:

Scores from Figure 8.2		Transformed Score
2 + 4 = 6/2	=	3.0
3 + 4 = 7/2	=	3.5
5 + 5 = 10/2	=	5.0
6 + 7 = 13/2	=	6.5
7 + 10 = 17/2	=	8.5
9 + 10 = 19/2	=	9.5

Step 2. Next, the autocorrelation coefficient is computed according to the procedure previously described for the transformed scores. It is noteworthy that in computation of the new autocorrelation coefficient for the transformed data, the number of data points is markedly reduced with use of the moving average transformation. In the present example, the data points are reduced from 12 to 6. The new autocorrelation coefficient computed with use of the transformed scores is .45. This coefficient is not significant

as determined by Bartlett's test ($2/\sqrt{6} = .82$). Therefore, the therapist can conclude that the serial dependency in the data set has been substantially reduced.

Figure 8.4 presents the original data series and the transformed data. The graph clearly shows how the moving average transformation "smoothed" out the data in the process of minimizing the autocorrelation. One obvious limitation of the moving average approach is that it reduces the number of data points in the process of transformation to approximately half of the original data points (see Figure 8.4*B*). This may be a serious limitation when the original number of data points is relatively small. Remember that Bartlett's test, which is part of the procedure for determining the significance of an autocorrelation coefficient, is not a valid test if 5 or fewer data points are used in computing the autocorrelation coefficient.

Once the serial dependency in a data series has been reduced, the therapist may proceed with whatever analytic procedure has been selected. In the remaining sections of this chapter, we discuss several of the more easily computed statistical procedures used in analyzing single system data. Before this, however, one last cautionary note regarding data transformations is in order. As stated previously, any data transformation will invariably modify the nature of a data series and result in a loss of some information which may be of value to the therapist and client. This should be kept in mind when transformations are performed. Also, if data are transformed for any phase of the data series, that transformation must be continued or extended to all the data points in the series. It is inappropriate and misleading to compare transformed data for one phase with nontransformed data from another phase in the same data series. Finally, there are numerous other data transformation procedures available (McCain and McCleary, 1979). The two presented in this chapter were selected for their computational ease. The first difference and moving average transformation procedures require only minimal mathematical skills and can easily be performed by therapists who are interested in comprehensively and systematically analyzing the data they collect to assess client performance.

STATISTICAL AND SEMISTATISTICAL PROCEDURES

Statistical methods of analyzing data collected from single system designs are being applied with increasing frequency (Kratochwill and Brody, 1978). A large number of methods are available and new methods and applications are being proposed at a fairly rapid rate (Edington, 1982; Tryon, 1982; Wolery and Billingsley, 1982). Some of these tests are

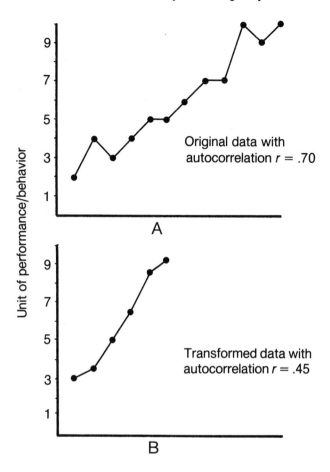

Figure 8.4. Line graphs showing original data series (*graph A*) and transformed data series (*graph B*). Data transformation was achieved by use of the integrated moving average procedure.

complex and esoteric, while others place only minimal demands on the statistical knowledge required by the user. Some authors (Gentile et al., 1972) have proposed that new statistical procedures are not necessary to analyze single system data. Instead, they argue, adaptations of conventional statistical procedures such as analysis of variance (ANOVA) and *t* tests are appropriate for use with single system data. The advantage of *t* tests and analysis of variance are that they are widely familiar to clinicians and researchers whose training has emphasized group-comparison designs. The primary criticism leveled against the use of conventional statistical procedures is related to the issue of serial dependency discussed in the previous section. Conventional parametric statistical procedures such as the t and F tests require that certain assumptions be met before they can be validly applied. One of the assumptions is that the data are independent. When there is serial dependency, the independence assumption is violated and t and F ratios do not follow the distribution from which inferences are generally made, which makes the use of the tests questionable (Hartman, 1974; Michael, 1974).

The assumption of independence for t and F tests refers to the independence of error components or to the correlation between the error components of a pair or series of observations. The expected value of the correlation between error components of observations is assumed to be zero. As shown in the previous section, this is typically not the case in data from single system designs in which there usually is some degree of serial dependency. Serial dependency can be reduced by the use of a transformation procedure, and some authors (Jayaratne and Levy, 1979) have suggested that once this is done, or if the autocorrelation coefficient for a data series is nonsignificant, the use of conventional statistical procedures may be permissible. A nonsignificant autocorrelation coefficient or reduction of serial dependency through data transformation, however, does not solve all the problems associated with the use of conventional statistical procedures. Analysis of variance and t tests are used to evaluate performance across phases or conditions by comparison of mean values. As discussed in Chapter 7, a problem with use of mean values as the basis of a comparison is that trends in the data are ignored. Ignoring trends makes statistical conclusions based on mean values difficult to interpret. For example, Figure 8.5 depicts an accelerating linear trend beginning at baseline and continuing through the intervention period. If the mean values for the baseline and intervention data were statistically compared with use of a t test, a significant difference would be revealed. The graph clearly indicates, however, that the linear trend in the data was a naturally occurring one and that the treatment had no effect. Conversely, if a t test were applied to the data presented in Figure 8.6, no significant difference between baseline and intervention phases would be revealed, since the mean level of performance in each phase is identical. Visual inspection of the data in Figure 8.6 clearly indicates, however, that the introduction of intervention produced a marked treatment effect, as indicated by the reversal in trend across the two phases.

Finally, the computation of conventional statistical procedures assumes a moderate degree of familiarity with statistical concepts and procedures. Therapists who do not have this moderate degree of statistical skill and, therefore, must rely on outside individuals or resources to help them compute quantitative procedures are not likely to use those procedures in the routine evaluation of client performance.

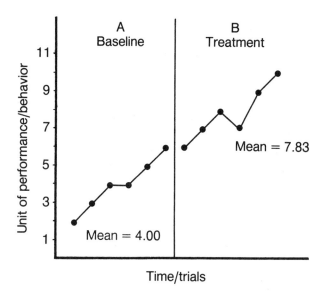

Figure 8.5. Line graph comparing data series and means for baseline and treatment phases.

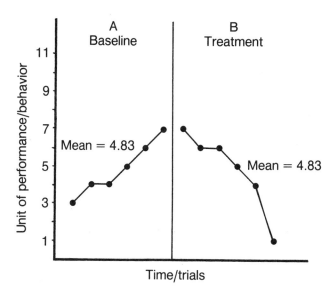

Figure 8.6. Line graph comparing data series and means for baseline and intervention phases.

The procedures presented in the remainder of this chapter may be considered semistatistical or what Jayaratne and Levy (1979) call "statistical rules of thumb." These procedures are specifically designed as judgmental aids for use with single system data. They require very little background in mathematics or statistics, and any graduate of an accredited baccalaureate program in occupational or physical therapy should be able to understand and compute them with relative ease. The weakness of the procedures is that the statistical properties of the methods have not been widely investigated and formal or sophisticated mathematical models justifying their use are not available. As noted previously, however, the procedures should be viewed as judgmental aids designed to provide a degree of quantitative confidence to the results obtained through graphic analysis and visual inspection.

Statistical Analysis and the Celeration Line Approach

As described in Chapter 7, the celeration line approach, also referred to as the "split-middle method," is a procedure designed to aid in the visual analysis of a trend in a client's response pattern. Use of the procedure results in the development of a celeration line or trend line indicating whether the baseline data are accelerating, decelerating, or stationary (see Figures 7.17, 7.18, and 7.19). As also noted, the celeration line computed for the baseline data should be extended into the intervention phase to predict client performance. The assumption made in extending the celeration line into the intervention phase is that if the treament has no effect, the client's response pattern will remain the same during intervention as during the baseline. In other words, the trend during baseline will continue during intervention. If the trend line in baseline divides the data points in half; i.e., half the data points fall above or on the celeration line and half the data points fall on or below the celeration line, the same pattern should occur in the intervention phase. This assumes, of course, that the intervention had no effect. If the intervention does produce a change in client performance during the intervention period, the proportion of data points either above or below the celeration line will change as a reflection of the change in client performance. This change in the proportion of data points provides the basis for a statistical comparison of client performance across the two phases.

An example will serve to illustrate the use of the celeration line approach to determine a statistical probability statement regarding client performance. Figure 8.7 displays the data series for a client's performance which was evaluated with use of a simple AB design. The celeration line has been computed for the baseline data with use of the procedures

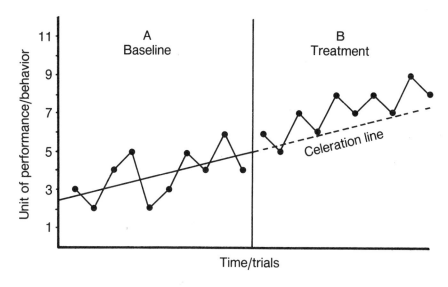

Figure 8.7. Line graph illustrating response pattern and celeration line across baseline and treatment phases. The celeration line was computed for baseline data and was extended into the treatment phase.

described in Chapter 7. The celeration line appears as a *solid line* in the baseline phase and separates the baseline data into two equal halves, with 50% of the data points above the celeration line and 50% below the celeration line. The celeration line has been extended into the intervention phase of the design and appears as a *dashed line*. Again, the hypothesis that is being evaluated here is that there is no change in performance across phases. If this is the case, the slope of the celeration line should be the same during the intervention phase as during the baseline phase. Thus, 50% of the data points in the treatment phase should fall on or above the projected celeration line, and 50% should fall on or below the celeration line. Obviously, this was not the case in this particular example. The finding that the proportion of data points above (or below) the celeration line during the intervention phase is different from that during the baseline phase suggests a change in the client's response pattern during intervention. Two simple methods may be used to determine whether this change was "statistically significant." One method is to use the probability table presented by Bloom (1975). The other is to compute a simple binomial test to determine a probability statement related to the proportion.

A probability table to compute the significance of the change in client performance appears as Table 8.1. To use the table, the therapist must first determine values to use in entering the probability table. In the example

Table 8.1.
Number of Treatment Observations above (or below) the Celeration Line Which Are Required to Demonstrate a Statistically Significant Effect[a]

	Number of Treatment Observations														
Proportion during Baseline[b]	4	6	8	10	12	14	16	18	20	24	28	32	36	40	60
.10	3	3	3	4	4	4	5	5	5	6	7	7	8	8	11
.15	3	3	4	4	5	5	6	6	7	8	8	9	10	11	15
.20	3	4	5	5	6	6	7	8	8	9	10	11	12	13	18
.25	4	4	5	6	7	7	8	9	9	11	12	13	14	16	22
.30	4	5	6	6	7	8	9	10	10	12	13	15	16	18	25
.35	4	5	6	7	8	9	10	11	12	13	15	17	18	20	28
.40	4	5	6	8	9	10	11	12	13	15	16	18	20	22	31
.45	4	6	7	8	9	10	11	13	14	16	18	20	22	24	34
.50		6	7	9	10	11	12	13	15	17	19	22	24	26	37
.55		6	8	9	10	12	13	14	16	18	21	23	26	28	40
.60		6	8	9	11	12	14	15	17	19	22	25	27	30	43
.65			8	10	11	13	14	16	17	20	23	26	29	32	46
.70				10	12	13	15	17	18	21	24	28	31	34	49
.75					12	14	16	17	19	22	26	29	32	35	51
.80						14	16	18	20	23	27	30	34	37	54
.85									20	24	28	31	34	38	56
.90												32	36	40	58

[a]Adapted from: Bloom, M. (1975). *The paradox of helping: Introduction to the philosophy of scientific practice.* New York: Macmillan, p. 203. Determined by use of the one-tailed test; $p < .05$

[b]If the proportion of baseline observations above or below the celeration line does not appear in the table, use the next larger proportion.

presented in Figure 8.7, the goal is for the client's performance to increase. The therapist, therefore, should determine the proportion of observations during the baseline period that fall above the celeration line by dividing the number of data points above the line by the total number of baseline observations. In this case, 5 baseline observations fall above the celeration line and 10 data points are included in the baseline period, so the proportion is 5/10 or .50. This proportion will be used to determine where to enter the probability table on the left-hand margin under the boxhead, "Proportion during Baseline." In most cases in which the celeration line approach is used in conjunction with a probability table, .50 will be the value used, since one of the outcomes of developing a celeration line with use of baseline data is to divide the data points into equal halves.

The next step is to determine the total number of data points plotted during the intervention phase. This value is used to enter the horizontal row of Table 8.1. In the example (Figure 8.7), there are a total of 10 data points in the *intervention* phase. The therapist would locate the value of 10 under the boxhead, ''Number of Treatment Observations.'' Now look down the column until the cell value corresponding to the proportion in the left-hand column (.50) is located. The intersection of these two values (.50 in the left-hand column and 10 in the horizontal row) is 9. This cell value indicates the number of data points in the treatment phase that must be above the extended celeration line in order for there to be a statistically significant change in client performance across the phases at the .05 level. Since 9 of 10 data points in the example illustrated in Figure 8.7 are above the projected celeration line, the client change across phases is considered statistically significant ($p < .05$).

The combined application of the celeration line and Table 8.1 represents a directional (one-tailed) test of significance for client change. That is why the therapist must specify whether the client change is expected to increase or decrease relative to the baseline data. If the information in Table 8.1 is used in a post hoc manner to determine whether client performance has either increased or decreased, the probability level is raised to .10. Bloom (1975) presents additional tables that may be used to test the statistical significance of client change at other confidence levels.

If the therapist does not have access to a probability table, an alternative method to determine the statistical significance of client change is to use a simple binomial test (Kazdin, 1976; White, 1972). The formula for computing a statistical probability based on the binomial test is: $\binom{n}{x} p^n$, where n is the number of data points in the intervention phase, x is the number of data points above (or below) the projected celeration lines, and p is the probability of obtaining x data points above or below the projected celeration line (Siegel, 1956). In the previous example (Figure 8.7), n is equal to 10, x is equal to 9, and p was previously determined to be .50. That is, p represents the proportion expected by chance which will be 5 data points above (or below) the celeration line when a total of 10 data points are included in the intervention phase ($p = 5/10$ or .50). Substituting these values in the formula $\binom{10}{9}.50^{10}$ results in a statistical probability of $p < .05$.

The celeration line approach was developed primarily to display trend and describe the process of change across phases rather than to make inferential judgments. The use of the binomial test with trend data, in particular, has been criticized (cf. Kazdin, 1976). The probability table is more conservative than the binomial test and represents the best method to determine a quantitative index related to client change based on statistical probability when the celeration line procedure is used.

As noted in Chapter 7, the celeration line approach is most appropriately used to analyze changes in trend and slope across phases. A limitation of this approach is that it requires a minimum of 7 to 10 data points in the baseline phase to accurately determine the celeration line. In addition, the baseline and intervention phases should contain a relatively equal number of data points so that any extraneous influences have an equal opportunity to influence the outcome.

One distinct advantage of the celeration line method is that it incorporates trend in the baseline as a basis for "predicting" client performance in the intervention phase. As a result of this characteristic, Bloom and Fischer (1982, p. 447) argue that the "celeration line approach takes into account most kinds of serial dependency involved in autocorrelation." By approximating trend in the baseline during the computation of the celeration line, the directionality and serial dependency in the data are taken into consideration.

It should be noted that serial dependency is a complex phenomenon that involves more than simple autocorrelation between data points (Glass et al., 1975). Another component of serial dependency, not previously discussed, is related to cyclical fluctuations or influences in the data series. The celeration line approach does not reduce or address this component of serial dependency. Huitema and Girman (1978) have demonstrated, however, that cyclic fluctuations are not common in data series routinely collected in clinical studies.

Overall, the celeration line represents an excellent method of quantitatively analyzing data from single system designs. The procedure is easy to compute, intuitively appealing, applicable to a large number of evaluations conducted in clinical environments, and particularly appropriate for analysis of client response patterns that evidence changes in trend across phases.

Two Standard Deviation Band Method

A second semistatistical approach or "statistical rule of thumb" that can be used to analyze single system data is the two standard deviation band method. This method of analysis assumes normally distributed data and should not be used with a data series that exhibits a significant autocorrelation coefficient. Once the serial dependency has been reduced to a nonsignificant level, the two standard deviation band method may be applied with a relatively high degree of statistical confidence. One advantage of this procedure is that it can be applied when there are a small number of data points in the baseline (5 to 10). Remember that one of the limitations of the celeration line approach is that a small number of baseline observations reduces the accuracy of the trend line computed from baseline data. The key to the two standard deviation band method is the computation of the standard deviation for the baseline data. Statistical significance is computed directly from the standard deviation of the scores. Thus, the central factor in applying this approach is the scores themselves rather than the number of observations. The steps employed in computing the two standard deviation band procedure follow.

Step 1. The data presented in Figure 8.7 and used to compute the celeration line approach have been reproduced in Figure 8.8 so that results from the two methods can be compared. The first step is to sum all the scores contained in the baseline: $3 + 2 + 4 + 5 + 2 + 3 + 5 + 4 + 6 + 4 = 38$.

Step 2. Then, square each of the values in the baseline and add them: $3^2 + 2^2 + 4^2 + 5^2 + 2^2 + 3^2 + 5^2 + 4^2 + 6^2 + 4^2 = 160$.

Step 3. Next, square the value obtained in the first step (38) divide this squared value by the number of observations ($n = 10$) in the baseline period:

$$(38)^2 = 1,444$$
$$1,444/10 = 144.4$$

Step 4. Next, subtract the result obtained in step 3 (144.4) from the result obtained in step 2 (160) and divide the resulting value by $n - 1$, where n equals the number of baseline observations.

$$\frac{\text{Value from Step 2} - \text{Value from Step 3}}{160 \qquad - \qquad 144.4} = 15.6$$

Then

$$15.6/(10 - 1) = 15.6/9 = 1.73$$

This new value (1.73) is the variance of the baseline scores.

Step 5. Then, take the square root of the value obtained in step 4, to determine one standard deviation.

$$\sqrt{1.73} = 1.32$$

The new value of 1.32 is one standard deviation.

Step 6. Next, compute the mean for the baseline scores by dividing the sum of the baseline scores obtained in step 1 by the total number of baseline scores (n).

$$\text{Mean} = 38/10 = 3.8$$

Step 7. Now draw two horizontal lines above and below the mean on the y-axis so that each line is two standard deviations from the mean. These lines are the boundaries of the two standard deviation band.

$$2 \text{ Standard Deviations} = 2 \times 1.32 = 2.64$$

The upper band is drawn at $3.8 + 2.64 = 6.44$. The lower band is drawn at $3.8 - 2.64 = 1.16$

Gottman and Leiblum (1974) argue that if at least two successive observations during the intervention phase (B) fall outside the two standard deviation band, a statistically significant change in client performance has occurred across the two phases. This statistical significance is based on the assumption that the likelihood of such an event occurring is less than 5 in 100 (Gottman and Leiblum, 1974; Jayaratne and Levy, 1979).

In the previous example (Figure 8.8), there are two or more successive data points in the intervention phase that fall above the plus two standard deviation (+ 2 S.D.) band, which indicates that a statistically significant change in performance has occurred across the two phases. Thus, both the celeration line approach and the two standard deviation band method demonstrate a statistically significant change for the same set of data (see Figure 8.7 and 8.8). As noted previously, one limitation of the two standard deviation band method is that it is sensitive to serial dependency in the data series. If there is a statistically significant degree of autocorrelation, the two standard deviation band method may not produce accurate results. Prior to using this approach, the therapist should determine the degree of autocorrelation in the data series. If there is a nonsignificant degree of autocorrelation, the two standard deviation band method may be applied directly to the data series. If, however, a significant autocorrelation coefficient is revealed, a data transformation technique such as the first difference transformation or the moving average transformation should be

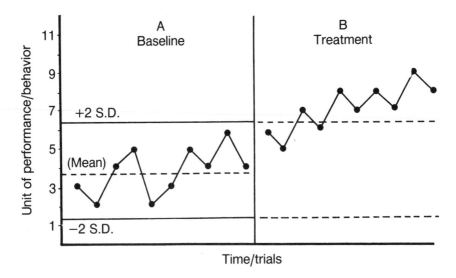

Figure 8.8. Line graph depicting the two standard deviation (*S.D.*) band procedure for determining statistical significance.

used to reduce the degree of serial dependency prior to computation of the two standard deviation band method.

One of the advantages of the two standard deviation band procedure is that it can be used with relatively small baselines. This is because the computation of the standard deviation and, therefore, the two standard deviation band takes into account the actual number of baseline observations. An increased variability in estimating the "true" level of baseline performance is reflected in a large standard deviation and, consequently, a larger two standard deviation band width outside which the client's performance must occur in order for change to be considered statistically significant. Therefore, the two standard deviation band method may be applied to baseline data that are fluctuating or evidencing a high degree of variability. This variability will be translated into a wider band of performance that will be used as the basis of comparison for performance during the intervention period (Bloom and Fischer, 1982).

C Statistic

Recently, Tryon (1982, p. 423) described the C statistic and argued that it provided a "simple, yet elegant method of time-series analysis that can be used on small data sets to evaluate the effects of treatment interventions." The C statistic can be applied to a data series with as few as eight observations and also can be applied to a data series that exhibits serial dependency (Tryon, 1982). The C statistic is used initially to evaluate baseline data. If the baseline data are found to contain a nonsignificant trend, the baseline and intervention data are combined and the C statistic is again computed to determine whether a statistically significant change has occurred. If the baseline data are found to contain a statistically significant trend, the C statistic can still be applied to the data by constructing a comparison data series, but its usefulness is more limited in this case (cf. Blumberg, 1984). The following steps are involved in computation of the C statistic.

Step 1. Assume that the data series illustrated in Figure 8.9 has been recorded for a client receiving therapy services. Obtain a difference score by subtracting the first score from the second, the second from the third, the third from the fourth, and so on, until all the scores are used. As noted previously, the C statistic is first computed for only the baseline data to determine whether there is a significant trend in that phase of the data series. In the example, only the 10 baseline data points are included in the calculations at this point: $2 - 2 = 0; 2 - 3 = -1; 3 - 5 = -2; 5 - 3 = 2; 3 - 4 = -1; 4 - 1 = 3; 1 - 3 = -2; 3 - 2 = 1; 2 - 5 = -3$.

Step 2. Next, square each of the values obtained in step 1 and add these squared values: $(0)^2 + (-1)^2 + (-2)^2 + (2)^2 + (-1)^2 + (3)^2 + (-2)^2 + (1)^2 + (-3)^2 = 33$. Note that since pairs of scores were used in step 1, there is one less value than the total number of baseline data points.

Step 3. The mean value for the baseline data points is computed by adding all the scores together and dividing by the total number of scores (n): $2 + 2 + 3 + 5 + 3 + 4 + 1 + 3 + 2 + 5 = 30/10 = 3$. The mean for this group of baseline scores is 3.

Step 4. Next, calculate a mean difference value for each score by subtracting each raw score from the mean value and then squaring the difference score. The sum of these squared mean difference scores is then obtained.

Baseline Score	−	Mean (Step 3)	=	Mean Difference	Mean Difference Squared
2	−	3	=	− 1	1
2	−	3	=	− 1	1
3	−	3	=	0	0
5	−	3	=	+ 2	4
3	−	3	=	0	0
4	−	3	=	+ 1	1
1	−	3	=	− 2	4
3	−	3	=	0	0
2	−	3	=	− 1	1
5	−	3	=	+ 2	4
				Sum	16

Step 5. The sum of the mean difference scores squared (16), which was obtained in step 4, is multiplied by 2 ($2 \times 16 = 32$).

Step 6. The values obtained in step 2 and in step 5 are inserted in the following formula:

$$C = 1 - \frac{\text{Step 2}}{\text{Step 5}}$$

$$C = 1 - \frac{33}{32}$$

$$C = 1 - 1.031$$

$$C = .031$$

The minus sign can be ignored in this step.

Step 7. Next, compute the standard error for the C statistic with use of the following formula:

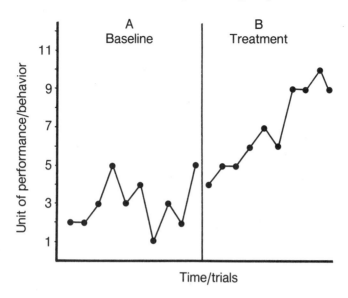

Figure 8.9. Line graph showing data series for baseline and treatment phases. The data were used to compute the *C* statistic.

$$\text{Standard Error} = \sqrt{\frac{n - 2}{(n - 1)(n + 1)}}$$

where *n* equals the number of scores in the data series for which the *C* statistic is being computed. In this case, $n = 10$.

$$\text{Standard Error} = \sqrt{\frac{8}{9(11)}} = .284$$

Step 8. For a determination of whether the *C* statistic is significant, a *Z* score is computed by dividing the *C* statistic value obtained in step 6 by the standard error obtained in step 7.

$$Z = \frac{\text{Step 6}}{\text{Step 7}}$$

$$Z = \frac{.031}{.284}$$

$$Z = .11$$

For any data series with 8 or more data points, a Z of 1.64 or more is statistically significant at a level of $p < .05$. This is a one-tailed test which means that the anticipated direction of the trend should be established prior to computing the statistic. Obviously, the Z value of .11 is less than the required value of 1.64 indicating that no significant trend exists in the baseline data. Once it has been established that a significant trend does not exist in the baseline, the therapist can then go on to compute a C statistic for the entire data series. That is, the data for the baseline and the intervention period are combined, and the eight steps outlined above are repeated with the entire data series. The C statistic computed for all 20 observations (baseline and intervention) displayed in Figure 8.9 is .820 and the standard error is .212. With use of the formula in step 8, the Z value for the entire data series is computed to be 3.87. This value exceeds the Z of 1.64 and suggests a statistically significant trend across baseline and intervention phases.

The C statistic is an easy-to-compute quantitative index that may prove useful to some clinicians. The primary advantage of the C statistic is that it can be computed for data that exhibit serial dependency. Tryon (1982) argues that autocorrelation will not adversely influence the results of the C statistic. Another definite advantage is that the C statistic can be computed for a data series with as few as eight observations or scores.

The C statistic is most useful when the baseline data are not found to be exhibiting a statistically significant trend, as in the previous example. When the first application of the C statistic to the baseline data indicates no significant trend, the data points from the intervention phase can legitimately be added to the baseline phase and the C statistic calculated to determine whether a significant change in performance exists across phases. If, on the other hand, the baseline data evidence a statistically significant trend when the C statistic is first computed with only baseline observations, it is not appropriate to add intervention and baseline scores together. If a significant trend exists in baseline, one possible solution is to compute a celeration line for the baseline data as described in Chapter 7. Once the celeration line is computed for the baseline phase, scores in the intervention phase are subtracted from the corresponding trend line values to form a new "data series." This comparison data series is then tested for trends with use of the C statistic. Another less powerful alternative method that can be used if a significant Z value is found for the baseline score is to subtract the corresponding data points in the baseline phase from those in the intervention phase to create a new data series which may be tested with the C statistic. The C statistic when used with either of the above alternative procedures is limited, since it will not be significant when the slopes of the data series in the two phases are relatively equal, but a dramatic change in level has occurred. This limitation may affect the interpretation of the results and should be considered whenever the C statistic is used with a data series in which the baseline scores have been shown to demonstrate a statistically significant trend.

The three statistical procedures presented in this chapter should provide the therapist with all the quantitative procedures necessary to evaluate the majority of data collected in clinical practice. The celeration line approach and the two standard deviation band method are extremely simple to compute, which thus enhances their heuristic and practical value. The C statistic is slightly more complex but requires only a minimum statistical background. Together, these statistical rules of thumb provide the therapist with predictive, quantitative methods that are easy to use and help to provide clinical direction by establishing a statistical basis for considering treatment to be either successful or ineffective. In fact, one of these three precedures should suffice as the preferred method of quantitative analysis for the vast majority of clinically based evaluations. Many other more sophisticated or specialized statistical procedures are available to analyze data from single system designs (Edington, 1980, 1982; Gottman and Glass, 1978; Kazdin, 1976; Johnston and Pennypacker, 1980), and the reader interested in pursuing the quantitative analysis of data collected from single system designs should consult these references.

— ADVANTAGES OF STATISTICAL ANALYSIS —

As noted previously, the use of statistical procedures can be particularly informative when new methods of intervention or programming are being evaluated. The effects associated with new and undeveloped programs or treatments are likely to be small and may not be considered therapeutically valuable if analyzed on a purely visual basis. The detection of small treatment effects would seem to be particularly important in fields such as occupational and physical therapy in which many of the treatment strategies are not well developed and in which there is often little opportunity to control many of the extraneous factors or variables that may function to limit or reduce treatment effectiveness. When these factors are considered along with the marked variability and heterogeneity associated with many of the disorders and conditions encountered in therapy settings, the argument could easily be made that small treatment effects would be the rule rather than the exception in the evaluation of clinically based interventions. Statistical procedures applied as adjuncts to visual inspection can help a therapist determine when a treatment effect has occurred and, perhaps more importantly, may help therapists to begin to identify and define some factors and variables associated with treatment success. If these factors or variables can be recognized, they may be manipulated or modified to enhance the effectiveness of intervention.

Another advantage associated with statistical analysis is related to the consistency of the results obtained by applying statistical procedures to a data series. It has been demonstrated that one of the weaknesses associated witn visual inspection is an inconsistent interpretation of the data across examiners or raters. Different people may look at the same graphs of performance and come to contrasting or contravening conclusions about the effectiveness of the treatment (DeProspero and Cohen, 1979; Gottman and Glass, 1978). In contrast to the inconsistency associated with a strict visual interpretation, results obtained via statistical procedures are extremely stable. If the computations are performed accurately, a given data series will produce the same quantitative result regardless of who does the calculations.

A final advantage associated with the use of statistical procedures is that they provide an objective method of validating the results obtained from visual analysis. In most cases, the results of statistical procedures will concur or confirm those obtained by visual inspection, which thus lends an added degree of quantitative confidence to the empirical findings.

DISADVANTAGES OF STATISTICAL ANALYSIS

One commonly cited disadvantage of employing statistical procedures with single system designs is related to the nature of the designs and the purpose of idiographic procedures. The logic associated with traditional quantitative procedures is to treat within-subject variability as ''error'' and to statistically control or reduce this variability (Sidman, 1960). One of the goals of single system strategies is to study intersubject and intrasubject variability as an integral component of the client change process. Single system designs allow therapists to evaluate functional relationships between behavior and environmental conditions that may contribute to variability. If excessive variability appears to be affecting treatment results, the clinician is encouraged to search for the source of the variability in a systematic manner and to manipulate it to the client's advantage. Statistical tests are criticized because they artificially control variability and thereby prevent the clinician from discovering important information related to client performance.

Another disadvantage of using quantitative procedures is that clinicians may begin to place undue faith in a statistical value and allow the statistical tests to make inferential dec. ions regarding the client's performance (Carver, 1978; Greenwald, 1975). Bakan (1966) has observed that investigators in the behavioral science often ''operationalize'' the inferential process by reporting the results of statistical tests. The use of statistical procedures and significance tests removes from the investigator the burden of making inferential decisions and transfers the responsibility to the test of significance. Such a trend would have obviously negative consequences for the evaluation of individual client performance.

A final objection to the use of statistical procedures has been outlined by Michael (1974). He argues that statistical procedures result in a collapsing or dichotomization of the evaluation process. The use of statistical methods may lead therapists to interpret the results of treatment as significant or nonsignificant. Such a judgment would de-emphasize the value of interpreting the client's pattern of responses during the various phases of the design. One of the strengths of the single system approach is that it emphasizes the study and evaluation of the intervention *process*. With a reliance on statistical significance, the therapist tends to ignore the therapeutic process and to focus instead strictly on therapeutic *outcomes*.

CONCLUSIONS

The use of statistical procedures to analyze data from single system designs is sure to increase (Kratochwill and Brody, 1978; Bloom and Fischer, 1982; Kazdin, 1982). If statistical procedures are used as adjuncts to visual analysis, as is suggested by Elashoff and Thoreson (1978), a substantial contribution to the evaluation process can be made. The three semistatistical procedures described in this chapter can provide the therapist with easy to use judgmental aids designed to facilitate data interpretation. One of the major advantages of the celeration line approach and the two standard deviation band method is that they cannot be computed without heavy reliance on graphic and visual procedures. Graphing of all of the scores or observations in a data series is an integral component of the analytic process for both of these methods. Thus, the therapist is required to combine both graphic and visual inspection in the use of the celeration line and two standard deviation band method. The C statistic can be computed with use of only the numeric values, without any graphic representation. It is strongly recommended that all three of the statistical rules of thumb presented in this chapter always be used in conjunction with graphic analysis and visual inspection of the data.

The statistical procedures presented in this chapter are all relatively new and untested. Each of the procedures should be considered an "approximate" method of analyzing data. They should be used only in conjunction with visual and graphic analysis, and therapists should be careful not to overinterpret the results of a statistical analysis.

CHAPTER 9

Single System Strategies: Summing Up

INTRODUCTION

The ultimate purpose of applied research in occupational and physical therapy is to develop and establish intervention techniques that can be successfully incorporated into clinical practice. The single system strategies presented in previous chapters are specifically designed to help therapists achieve the goal of developing a scientifically respected practice. The primary purpose of single system evaluation designs is to evaluate treatment effectiveness and document clinically significant improvements in client performance. From a practical standpoint, the cost of implementing and coordinating client evaluation is small. Several single system designs, such as the multiple baseline design, can be initiated in most clinical environments with little or no disruption to routine therapeutic activities. Single system methods represent a systematic unobtrusive way to document the therapeutic effectiveness of ongoing intervention with a specific client and, simultaneously, to satisfy accountability needs. This strength of single system procedures is particularly important in view of the growing demand by third party payers for objective documentation of the benefits of therapy services.

Some therapists using single system methods will be interested in going beyond the documentation of clinical effectiveness for a specific client. The logical extension of single system procedures involves attempts to generalize the findings beyond the individual client or specific treatment setting. Furlong and Wampold (1981) identified four basic questions that therapists must answer before making inferences regarding treatment effectiveness that go beyond the documentation of client performance: (1) Are the data and findings reliable? (2) Was the alteration in the client's performance due to the intervention? (3) Was the change in performance significant or meaningful? (4) Are the results generalizable to other individuals and/or settings? The first two questions deal with the internal validity of the evaluation procedures and the last two questions relate to evaluation across studies and external validity.

The issues of internal and external validity as related to single system designs are briefly dealt with in Chapter 3. The discussion begun in Chapter 3 is expanded here. The reader may wish to refer back to Chapters 2 and 3 to review briefly the terminology and discussion of the issues concerning internal and external validity.

INTERNAL VALIDITY

White (1984) argues that single system designs are no more jeopardized by threats to internal validity than are traditional group-comparison designs. Those threats to internal validity which are controlled for by random assignment to groups in the traditional large-N designs (e.g., history, maturation, testing, instrumentation, statistical regression, and selection) are similarly controlled for in single system designs by the multiple application and withdrawal of the intervention and by the use of repeated measures or alterations in phases across clients, settings, or behaviors (Hacker, 1980; Levy and Olson, 1979; Tawney and Gast, 1984). As discussed in Chapter 3, the use of repeated measures does require the therapist to be especially aware of the possible confounding influence of testing and instrumentation effects. The use of valid and reliable measures to determine outcome effects in combination with the sequential application and withdrawal of the program appears to provide adequate control over these two frequently cited threats to the internal validity of single system designs (Kazdin, 1982).

Kratochwill (1978) provides a detailed discussion of how well specific single system designs control for the traditional threats to internal validity identified by Campbell and Stanley (1963). In addition to these ''classic'' threats, several other possible confounds have been identified with specific implications for single system designs.

Cycling Behavior

One of the distinguishing characteristics of single system strategies is that information on the client's performance is repeatedly collected over an extended period of time. That data are collected over time introduces the possibility that temporal cycles in the client's behavior may influence the results. The possibility of cycling behavior would appear to pose more of a problem for single system designs than for traditional group-comparison designs in which data are generally collected infrequently, over a much shorter period of time. Introduction and withdrawal of an intervention program will possibly coincide with a natural cycle in behavior or performance, which will result in the appearance of a functional relationship between treatment and outcome measures when, in fact, the effect was the result of some cyclic event. As an illustration, suppose that a patient with severe depression was admitted to a state mental hospital. After a period of time the patient was enrolled in an occupational therapy treatment program. The therapist began to measure some overt behavior related to the client's depression such as the number of verbal contacts with other clients during each therapy session and noticed a marked improvement in the patient's interactions with other clients. Suppose that this increase in verbal contacts coincided with the introduction of new treatment that coincidentally was introduced in April when the season was changing. It may be that the patient's depression was cyclic in nature and that he tended to spontaneously recover in the spring. If the therapist was unaware of this cyclic component of the client's behavior, he or she may have misinterpreted the client's improvement as due to the introduction of the new treatment program. Fortunately, there are a number of safeguards against the confounding influence of cyclic behavior. First, multiple applications and withdrawals of the program can be made. With each additional application and withdrawal of the program it becomes less likely that cyclic performance would consistently be associated with every application and withdrawal of the intervention. Second, a combination of ABA and multiple baseline designs can be employed. In such a combination, cyclic behavior would be expected to be reflected across the phases, including the treatment and baseline periods.

Statistical Conclusion Validity

Cook and Campbell (1979) identified statistical conclusion validity as a possible threat to the validity of traditional group-comparison designs. Statistical conclusion validity basically refers to the issue of design and analysis sensitivity. If the evaluation procedures are not sufficiently sensitive to uncover a presumed relationship between intervention and outcome measures, there may be a threat to statistical conclusion validity.

This threat was originally identified by Campbell (1969) as a threat to internal validity and was referred to as instability. Cook and Campbell (1979) have elaborated statistical conclusion validity into a separate category or group of threats, the majority of which deal with the power (sensitivity) of statistical and design manipulations. In our discussion, we consider statistical conclusion validity to be a type of threat to internal validity.

Statistical procedures provide the quantitative criterion by which the results of traditional group-comparison designs are judged. If statistical procedures are not applied in single system evaluations, the argument may be made that the power or sensitivity of the analysis is low and will not detect a functional relationship between the intervention and outcome measure. That is, how can a therapist accurately and consistently distinguish between a highly reliable treatment effect and one that may have occurred by chance? As noted in Chapter 7, there is evidence indicating that what looks like a clinically significant change (based on visual inspection) to one examiner may not be interpreted as clinically significant by another (DeProspero and Cohen, 1979; Gottman and Glass, 1978; Furlong and Wampold, 1982).

The argument against the use of statistical procedures to analyze single system data charges that if a therapeutic effect is so small that it requires the application of statistical tests to determine whether a change has occurred, the clinical significance of such an intervention is suspect. Thus, it has been asserted that the reliability of a given treatment effect lies in the ability to replicate clear and marked control over the outcome measure of interest and not in artificially or statistically inflating subtle treatment effects (Parsonson and Baer, 1978).

As noted in Chapter 8, there is an increasing trend toward the application of quantitative procedures with single system designs. Those who advocate the use of quantitative statistical methods argue that while clear and unequivocal effects need not be subjected to statistical analyses, there are situations in which visual inspection alone is not adequate. In particular, they argue further, statistical analysis can be helpful in evaluating the data from single system designs in which there is a significant degree of serial dependency (Jones et al., 1978).

Jones et al. (1977) have argued that the criteria used in making visual inferences from single system data are statistical in nature. That is, the components of visual analysis such as trend, variability and slope are statistical concepts. Therefore, inferences based on these concepts are based on statistical properties of the data collected from single system designs. Whether a therapist actually calculates a statistical test or relies on a visual appraisal of the data is irrelevant. The fact remains that the statistical properties of the data series form the basis for making judgments about treatment effectiveness. The point made by Jones et al. (1977) is that the difference between graphic analysis and visual inspection of single system evaluation data and statistical analysis of the same data are more apparent than real.

In a traditional group-comparison design, an intergroup statistical comparison is generally performed to determine whether the intervention produced a statistically significant treatment effect. In a single system design, an intrasubject comparison is performed to provide the same information. An example will serve to illustrate the similarities in the two procedures. The data for a hypothetical client receiving therapy appears in Figure 9.1. A typical AB design with a single baseline and intervention phase was used to collect the data. The therapist evaluating these data would look at the client's performance within each phase and across the two phases and make a judgment about the effectiveness of the intervention. The data display a small degree of variability within each phase (average fluctuations of 2 responses per trial between one trial and the next within each phase). There is, however, a marked change in level across the two phases (a difference of approximately 8 responses). After visually inspecting the data, the therapist is likely to conclude that the change occurring *between phases* is much greater than any change occurring *within a phase*. The data suggest that the intervention is resulting in a clinically significant treatment effect.

In a typical group-comparison design, a statistical test would take the place of the graphing and visual inspection. The statistical test, however, is essentially a comparison of the variation of scores *within a group* and variation of scores *between the groups*. Table 9.1 contains the same data as in Figure 9.1, with one important exception. The data in Table 9.1 are for two different groups rather than for two separate phases or conditions for the same client. In the calculation of a simple statistical test such as the *t* test or the *F* test, the mean scores for the two groups will be compared, with

Table 9.1.
Raw Scores for Two Groups of Subjects[a]

	Control Group	Treatment Group
	4	12
	7	14
	4	11
	6	15
	3	12
	6	14
	4	12
	6	14
Total	40	104
Mean	5	13
Standard deviation	1.41	1.41

[a] These data are the same as the data in Figure 9.1.

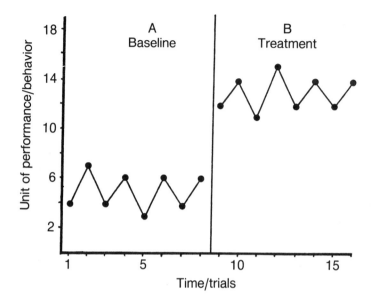

Figure 9.1. Data for a hypothetical client indicates a change in level of performance from baseline to intervention.

consideration given to the variability within each group and across the two groups. With use of the F test, a statistically significant value ($p < .05$) would be obtained which would indicate that the intervention produced a statistically significant treatment effect in the treatment group compared with the control group.

The above example, it is hoped, illustrates that the analytic logic behind the two procedures is essentially the same. The difference lies mainly in the choice of a criterion for determining whether the variation within groups or conditions and the variation between groups or conditions are significant. It should be emphasized, however, that traditional group-comparison designs and single system designs are not directly interchangeable. With use of group-comparison designs, there are questions posed about an intervention's average effect on a group of subjects. Inferences are then made concerning the average effect on the sample. Then, generalization is made to the population that the sample represents. The accuracy of the generalization to the target population depends on how well the population is represented by the sample.

Such generalizations cannot be made with use of single system strategies, since these designs neither attend to the average effects of interventions on groups nor use groups of subjects selected to represent a given population. Generalizations can be drawn from single system evaluation only when specific replication strategies, to be discussed in the next section, are used.

Overall, it appears that statistical analysis would help therapists to more sensitively and accurately judge the reliability of an intervention effect and to protect against statistical conclusion invalidity. With the use of statistical procedures, there is the possibility that some statistically significant but clinically insignificant effects will be reported. The obvious compromise, as recommended in Chapter 8, is for the therapist to report both the graphed data for visual inspection and the summarizing statistical analysis. Several reports in the therapeutic literature have used this strategy (cf. Ottenbacher, 1983; Ottenbacher et al., 1983; Ray et al., 1983). Performed together, statistical analysis and visual inspection of the data provide complementary information related to treatment impact and, thereby, enhance confidence in conclusions based on the data.

Order and Sequence Interactions

Kratochwill (1978) and White (1984) have discussed the possible threat of intervention sequence and order interactions. This threat to internal validity is more likely in single system designs than in the typical group-comparison design. As noted in Chapter 6, whenever a client is exposed to more than one intervention, there is the possibility that the effect of any one treatment is confounded with its order in the treatment sequence. The most common method of evaluating or controlling potential order or sequence effects in single system designs is to employ a design in which each condition is both preceded and succeeded by every other condition. If only baseline and a single intervention are being evaluated, a simple ABA design may be sufficient. When more than one treatment alternative is employed, however, the design becomes increasingly more complicated and more difficult to implement in the typical clinical environment. The careful scheduling of intervention and nonintervention alternating sequences can produce very strong evidence that order and sequencing effects are unlikely to account for the observed effects, particularly if shifts in performance are abrupt at the points of intervention.

Reactive Interventions

The threat of reactive interventions is a potential confound for single system designs. Kratochwill (1978, p. 16) has defined reactive intervention as intervention occurring when an investigator "intervenes into a data series as a reaction to either a past or [an] impending change in that series." For example, a therapist may implement a new treatment program for a client with rheumatoid arthritis in reaction to a sudden flare-up of the condition which results in increased joint pain and swelling. If, on initiation of the treatment, the client's pain recedes and the joint range of motion returns to the pretreatment level, the change or improvement may reflect a natural return to preintervention levels. This threat is similar to the regression phenomenon observed in group-comparison designs when subjects are selected because of extreme scores on a pretest (see Chapter 2). This threat is more common in a single system evaluation than in the traditional group-comparison design because more baseline information is generally available in a single system design. The temptation with use of a single system design is for the therapist to introduce the intervention at a time when the baseline data are evidencing extreme values.

One method to reduce the effect of reactive interventions as a threat to internal validity is to predetermine the length of each phase prior to the actual implementation of the design. The disadvantage of this approach is that the baseline or other phases cannot be maintained until a stable response pattern is obtained. Predetermining the length of phases also reduces the flexibility of the design, which is one of the major advantages of the single system approach. Kratochwill (1978) suggests that the evaluator using single system methods carefully examine the baseline data and avoid introducing the treatment at a point when the data series is evidencing any unusual or extreme increases or fluctuations.

As noted previously, several authorities argue that single system designs are at least as effective as group designs in determination of those aspects of an intervention that are responsible for treatment effects (Bloom and Fischer, 1982; Kazdin, 1982). Many potential threats to internal validity are reduced because only one client is often included in the design and serves as his or her own control. Additional control over possible confounds is derived from the repeated and frequent measures obtained for each client. This process allows the therapist to pinpoint more precisely when significant fluctuations in the dependent measure occur. This approach affords the therapist a much greater opportunity to detect potential sources of invalidity and to address them directly or to determine the impact that they might have on the intervention being evaluated.

EXTERNAL VALIDITY

The results of a single system evaluation are considered externally valid when they are representative of the effects that can be achieved when the intervention is employed in different settings or with different clients. As noted in Chapter 3, the issue of generalizability is a complex one that is often misinterpreted.

Possible threats to internal validity can be controlled for as a function of the design used in both group-comparison studies and single system evaluations. Unfortunately, design modifications cannot control for threats to external validity in either paradigm. In the group-comparison approach, the generalizability of findings across individuals depends on the degree to which any study meets the fundamental assumption that the participants in the sample are representative of a given population. In theory, at least, this assumption is assured by the random selection of a sizable sample from a defined target population. As noted in previous chapters, however, random selection and random assignment of homogeneous groups of clients are rarely feasible in clinical settings.

The probability that random selection and assignment will be effective in reducing threats to external and internal validity, respectively, is directly related to the number of clients available and inversely related to the heterogeneity of the sample. The low incidence of and the marked heterogeneity in most handicapped populations would appear to argue against the effective use of random selection and assignment with these populations (Ottenbacher, 1984b). In addition, predicting generalizability of findings from group-comparison studies also assumes that the particular client or clients to whom findings are to be generalized will respond in the same manner as did the majority of the members of the sample rather than as those for whom the intervention was unsuccessful. Thus, successful predictions and replications of group-comparison studies remain elusive in applied fields concerned with the welfare and the treatment of disabled or handicapped individuals (Birnbauer, 1981; Epstein, 1980).

The issue of external validity of single system evaluation and research is addressed by employing a different frame of reference than that used in group-comparison research. Findings from single system evaluations gain generalizability across individuals and settings by employment of direct replications, systematic replication, and clinical replication. These components of generalizability which are described briefly in Chapter 3 are presented in detail next.

Direct Replication

Direct replication is usually achieved by an investigator replicating a study with several different clients under similar conditions. The advantage of this approach is that variability between individuals and the interaction between different subject characteristics and the intervention procedure can be examined closely due to the direct and continuous measurement of the outcome variable (Hersen and Barlow, 1976; Barlow and Hersen, 1984; Leitenberg, 1973). Systematic adjustments in the procedure can be made and examined under controlled conditions, which further adds to the cumulative knowledge of the limitations and generality of an intervention strategy.

Direct replication is closely tied to the reliability of the treatment procedures. That is, a treatment shown to be effective more often or more consistently is certainly a more reliable procedure (Kazdin, 1982). Moreover, direct replication is relevant to establishing the generality of a treatment to individuals with problems similar to those of the client currently being treated. Hersen and Barlow (1976) caution, however, that generality from direct replication is restricted to statements concerning the population studied. Generalizations about the effectiveness of the treatment when administered by other therapists or in other settings are not possible from direct replications.

Sidman (1960) divides direct replications into two basic categories: (1) replication of the same intervention on one client and (2) replication of an intervention on more than one client. Remember that single system designs have built into them one of these forms of replication. The first kind of direct replication proposed by Sidman (1960), repetition of the same intervention on one client, forms an integral component of any ABAB design. In this design, the second AB replicates the first. Repetition of baseline and treatment in an ABAB design adds reliable evidence that the treatment is effective if results from the second administration parallel those from the first.

Direct replication across other clients occurs outside the internal components of a design and is the most frequent form of replication used in single system evaluation and research. Hersen and Barlow (1976) have recommended that three replications in addition to the original demonstration of treatment effectiveness are adequate evidence of direct replication. Along this line, Denenberg (1978) has argued that, if an investigator was to have access to a sample of 50 cases and if at least 1 case yields a finding that replicates the original one, the probability that this occurred by chance alone is less than .05. If the sample has more than 50 cases but fewer than 350, the probability of finding two or more cases like the original one is less than .05. Direct replication with three clients, as recommended by Hersen and Barlow (1976), provides initial evidence that the evaluation finding was not due to chance.

Hersen and Barlow (1976) also specify that for direct replication to occur, the clients involved in each of the replications should be as similar as possible, the therapist should remain the same, and the setting should remain unchanged while the replications are being conducted.

Admittedly, obtaining homogeneous clients, particularly in handicapped populations, for direct replication is not always possible. Recognizing that all variables may not be taken into account, the therapist should attempt to match the clients as closely as possible in a direct replication series. Problems in matching may be compensated for partially by obtaining an exhaustive measure during baseline. If clients are matched closely on baseline performance, the therapist can at least feel confident that all clients performed similarly on the behavior of interest before the intervention was introduced, even if they differed on other characteristics.

Generalizability from direct replications allows the therapist to postulate the possible range of client variability for treatment success. Direct replication does not provide evidence on subject performance in the presence of other therapists or in other settings. Such evidence requires systematic replication.

Systematic Replication

Systematic replication consists of varying settings, therapists, clients, or conditions (disorders), either singly or in combination, to determine whether treatment continues to be effective when these variables are modified. The ultimate test of generalizability for any treatment finding is whether other therapists can implement the intervention procedure under other situational conditions with other clients and achieve similar outcomes. That is, an evaluation gains functional generalizability by systematic replication (Hersen and Barlow, 1976; Barlow and Hersen, 1984; Sidman, 1960). Systematic replications are required if broad evidence of the generalizability of intervention is desired. Systematic replications are essential to establishing the overall effectiveness of a treatment.

As noted previously, direct replication involves comparisons across several single system designs with a series of homogeneous clients. Systematic replication, on the other hand, compares the effect of a specific treatment across other behaviors, settings, clients, and therapists. Different clients may be involved in both direct and systematic replications. The difference is that in direct replication, clients are matched as closely as possible, while in systematic replication, diversity among clients is allowed and sometimes encouraged.

The amount of variation between clients is one factor that differentiates direct and systematic replication; classification of a replication as systematic or direct is not always easy, however. A therapist may select clients differing from each other on only one or two characteristics, on several characteristics, or totally.

Systematic replication is a built-in element in multiple baseline designs which are discussed in Chapter 6. One advantage of the multiple baseline design is increased generalizability. As noted in Chapter 6, a multiple baseline design may be employed across behaviors, across clients, or across settings. These are also the aspects varied in systematic replications. The only other factor that can be varied in systematic replications, but not in multiple baseline designs, is the therapist administering the intervention. Multiple baseline designs are an excellent starting point for systematic replications and provide a useful mechanism for demonstrating the generalizability of intervention effects.

Although multiple baseline designs may provide an initial step in beginning systematic replication, it must be recognized that obtaining generalizability through systematic replication is a long-term process. Systematic replications may continue over a period of time before the generalizability of a treatment effect can be established. Examples of long-term programs of systematic replication with use of single system procedures are not yet available in the rehabilitation fields. As single system procedures are more widely understood and employed by therapists, programs of systematic replication, it is hoped, will be developed.

Use of systematic replication will allow the therapist to go beyond the documentation of client progress and begin to establish the scientific legitimacy and clinical generalizability of various intervention procedures. The development of a systematic replication program will require that therapists document and disseminate the results of previous evaluations with their professional colleagues. Operational definitions of treatment and outcome measures and precise detailed descriptions of measurement procedures will be required if other therapists are to attempt systematic replication of a particular treatment finding (Birnbauer, 1981).

Clinical Replication

Hersen and Barlow (1976) define clinical replication as an ''advanced replication procedure'' in which related treatment procedures are applied to a series of clients with multiple disorders that cluster together into what is generally recognized as a diagnostic syndrome. Clinical replication occurs following direct replication or in conjunction with systematic replication efforts. In direct replication, the goal is to demonstrate a functional relationship between a specific treatment procedure and a specific outcome in a homogeneous series of clients. At this level of replication, one treatment procedure is applied to one well-defined problem in similar clients. In systematic replication the variability in the series of clients treated is increased. In addition, the settings, therapists, and outcome behaviors may be varied. Direct and systematic replication procedures are strategies more often concerned with establishment of the generalizability of a functional relationship between a specific procedure and a particular behavior. Often this relationship includes only one component of a treatment program as applied to isolated behaviors. With clinical replication, the issue of generalizability of a treatment ''package'' which consists of two or more related intervention procedures applied to a series of clients who demonstrate similar combinations or clusters of multiple disorders is addressed. Clinical replication emphasizes the replication of well-defined intervention or treatment programs for well-defined groups or clusters of clinically relevant problems with a large number of clients. For example, a clinical replication series might be designed to address the issues of effectiveness and generalizability of a group of treatment techniques associated with neurodevelopmental therapy for treatment of a cluster of disorders encountered in cerebral palsy. Obviously, clinical replication involves a complex, comprehensive series of single system studies. Hersen and Barlow (1976) refer to this process as "technique building" and characterize it as a systematic applied research effort which extends over a period of several years. Initially, single system strategies are used to study individual intervention programs in the technique-building stage. Later, group-comparison designs may be used to evaluate the entire intervention package; this process is referred to as technique testing.

No treatment programs in occupational or physical therapy have been evaluated with use of a clinical replication series, although there is the potential and the need for this type of evaluation. Developing a clinical replication series requires considerable planning, effort, and resources. The advantage of implementing such a series is the increased generalizability of and the increased confidence that a therapist can have in a treatment package that has been developed and validated with use of clinical replication.

SOCIAL VALIDATION

For true generalizability, treatment effects revealed in isolated evaluations of intervention programs must be assessed in a broader, more complex social context. Social validation provides a mechanism for determining whether client improvements are maintained and extended into the client's everyday environment. Social validation provides evidence of whether the effects observed in treatment situations are of value in the client's natural environment.

According to Kazdin (1982, pp. 19–20), social validation refers to whether the focus of the intervention and changes in behavior or performance resulting from treatment "meet the demands of the social community of which the client is a part." This general definition was adapted from Wolf (1978) who suggests there are three levels of social validation: goals, procedures, and effects. For the therapist, these translate into a limited series of questions. Is a desired "therapeutic" outcome really socially important in the client's environment? Is the intervention socially appropriate and the least intrusive, most efficient method available to produce the desired outcome? Finally, does the intervention result in a socially appreciable improvement in client performance?

In answering the first question, the therapist is dealing with the issue of social importance as it relates to the expected outcome of treatment. For example, the goal for a client who has suffered a stroke and has a deficit in visual perception and spatial orientation may be to complete a specially designed puzzle. This therapist-selected goal of successfully completing the puzzle may be directly related to perceptual function but may have low social validity. How important will it be for the client to perform this activity in his or her everyday natural environment? A different goal, such as successfully dressing, may have a much higher social validity and still be related to visual perceptual function. Kazdin (1977, 1982) has suggested two means of measuring or assessing the social validity of a treatment goal. The first is social comparison. Social comparison involves comparison of the client's performance to that of a peer group. The performance level of the peer group may be ascertained through observation or through normative data. The performance level of the client's peer group is used to determine the goals toward which the client should be working. When the client achieves this goal, he or she will be functioning in a manner similar to peers, and the peer group level of function is assumed to be representative of socially valued behavior.

The second method of determining the social appropriateness of the treatment goals is by subjective evaluation (Kazdin, 1977, 1982). Subjective evaluation involves soliciting the opinions or judgments of experts or persons familiar with the client. These persons are in a position to determine the client's need for treatment and can help define what the goals for treatment should be. Kazdin (1982) points out that many of the decisions regarding treatment goals involve the use of subjective evaluation on an informal basis. Parents, relatives, friends, professional colleagues, and others often are responsible for identifying when a client needs treatment and what the outcomes of that treatment should be. Subjective evaluation simply formalizes this process and helps ensure that the objective of achieving a level of client performance that is both functional and socially relevant is attained.

The second question deals with selecting a treatment strategy that is socially appropriate. This question concerns ethics as much as generalizability. Presumably, a client's satisfaction with a particular intervention procedure is critical in determining whether that procedure will be utilized or will have an enduring effect on client performance. Factors that affect a procedure's social validity are severity, cost, and appeal (Kazdin, 1982).

Severity refers to employment of less threatening and noninvasive interventions prior to consideration of those treatment approaches that may cause the client a degree of apprehension or discomfort. Along this same line, treatments that are less expensive should be attempted prior to those that may require considerable time and expense. Finally, interventions that are simple, straightforward, and readily understood by clients have greater social validity than those that are esoteric and appear to bear little relationship to the client's disorder or the goal established for treatment.

The final component of social validity which is identified by Wolf (1978) deals with the social relevance and significance of the treatment effect, and this concept of social validity is the most useful and widely applied. Kazdin (1977, 1982) argues that the same two methods used to assess the social validity of the treatment goal, that is, social comparison and subjective evaluation, can be employed to determine the social validity of the treatment effect.

In the use of social comparison to determine the social significance of a treatment effect, the performance of a client before and after intervention is compared with the performance of nonhandicapped peers who did not require treatment. If the client's performance falls within a normal range as defined by peer group performance, the treatment effect is considered socially valid. For social comparison, individuals judged competent in the performance of a particular skill are selected and their performance level is determined, or alternatively, predetermined normative standards already available are used (Van Houten, 1979). When the comparison is made with use of normative data, however, it may be made with the best or higher level performance of the nonhandicapped or norm group rather than with the average performance of this group.

The other method for measuring the social importance of a treatment effect is subjective evaluation. Subjective evaluation involves the use of judges to rate the client's performance both before and after treatments (Kazdin, 1977). The judges may be persons familiar with the client or may be experts identified by the therapist who are in a position to make a determination regarding the before and after level of client performance. Ratings by the judges may be confined to performance in a specific area, or they may be more global in nature and the issue of the client's overall ability to function in his or her environment may be addressed (Kazdin, 1982; Yeaton, 1982). Subjective evaluation is obviously susceptible to the introduction of bias on the part of the raters or judges. If the guidelines provided by Kazdin (1977, 1982), Wolf (1978), and others are followed, however, subjective evaluation may provide a valuable adjunctive method for documenting the clinical significance and social relevance of the treatment effects.

Social validation procedures have not been used by therapists to assist in establishing the *in vivo* usefulness of treatment. Although both the effectiveness of the treatment and its functional value are difficult for the clinician to document, the failure of therapists to employ social validation is unfortunate. Social validation procedures are not sufficient, in isolation, to demonstrate the effectiveness of a treatment procedure or to establish its generalizability, but they certainly represent a valuable adjunctive technique that should be employed with single system designs whenever this is possible.

_____ EVALUATION AND RESEARCH _____

The terms evaluation and research are used interchangeably throughout this text. This coalescing of the two terms was intentional and based on the conviction that single system evaluation strategies provide the ideal method for integrating research and practice. As Bloom and Fischer (1982, p. 16) note,

probably the most productive way of assessing whether or not our practice is successful is through the use of systematized, objective methods of research that are capable of being repeated (replicated) by others. This is the science of practice, and it involves any number of features: professional action, informed by the best possible information available at any given time, combined with objective evaluation components.

The advantage of treating evaluation and research synonymously is that it allows the clinician to become an active participant in the clinical research process and to legitimately assume the role of the ''scientific practitioner.'' Bloom and Fischer (1982, p. 18) state that ''single system designs provide a basis for the integration of research and practice in as systematic and purposeful a way as possible. This kind of integration is the one that we believe is most likely to enhance our chances of success with our clients and consumers.''

The emergence of a scientist-clinician who is able to integrate research and practice is certainly to be encouraged. The use of systematic objective evaluation procedures that are equated by therapists and others as clinical research may cause some potential problems, however. To make some distinctions between formal research and systematic evaluation is important. The use of formal designs and data analysis procedures may lead some therapists and administrators to view single system-based client evaluations as formal research.

On functional grounds, treatment research and treatment evaluation may be viewed quite differently. Although the techniques and procedures may be very similar, the goals and purposes of treatment _research_ and treatment _evaluation_ are different. Bloom and Fischer (1982) list the following methodological commonalities between research and evaluation: formulate the problem; review the literature; develop objectives and goals; define the outcome (dependent) variable; develop a design; define the treatment; collect data; analyze data; and report findings. These stages or steps are characteristic of both treatment evaluation and treatment research. Although the steps involved in both activities are similar, the goals are not

(Barlow et al., 1984). The underlying goal of research in the ''classical'' sense is to develop better organized theories or explanations of relationships between events. The goal of pure treatment, on the other hand, is to improve client function, and the goal of treatment evaluation is to document the improvement in client function. The distinction between treatment and research may be viewed as existing on a continuum. In ''pure'' treatment, the only goal is improved client performance. In treatment evaluation, the primary goal is related to improved client outcome, but the therapist would also like to identify some characteristics of the treatment associated with improvement. In treatment evaluation, there is a secondary emphasis on developing scientific inferences related to the intervention. The next point on the continuum is treatment research. In treatment research, the goal is primarily the understanding of the treatment process and how it works and how it is related to theory development. In treatment research, client improvement is secondary to developing a better understanding of the treatment and how it works. The client's specific needs are not the central concern; rather, the client's needs are accommodated within the research framework. Finally, in ''pure'' research, the only goal is the generation of knowledge and better or more accurate scientific statements related to the phenomenon under study. Client improvement in any direct sense is not even a secondary goal in ''pure'' research. The results of this type of research may eventually be translated into procedures that will benefit future clients, but the immediate goal is the testing of theory or the generation of scientifically validated principles or statements.

The majority of the discussion throughout the previous chapters of this text has assumed that the procedures described would be used primarily by therapists engaged in *treatment evaluation* activities. Treatment evaluation is basically a matter of adopting an empirical approach to treatment. The primary goal in treatment evaluation is the improvement of the client, and single system strategies are employed to monitor and document this improvement. The use of single system procedures in treatment evaluation will make interventions more systematic and provide better information to support clinical decision making. The generation of scientific statements or inferences related to treatment effectiveness and theory development are secondary goals in this process.

When the goal is treatment evaluation, single system procedures can be applied on a routine basis to all clients with whom the therapist comes into contact. If, on the other hand, the therapist's primary goal is *not* client improvement but is the generation of scientific information or testing of scientific hypotheses related to a particular treatment procedure, the therapist is conducting *treatment research*. In this case, the clients involved in the treatment research must be treated as research subjects and afforded the appropriate safeguards, such as informed consent. In both cases (treatment evaluation and treatment research), the same single system design and analysis procedures may be used, but the goals are substantially different. If a treatment is being used in order to study its merits and not because of the client's specific need, the enterprise becomes more formal treatment research and not treatment evaluation, and the full protections given human subjects involved in research studies are required.

The perspective taken throughout this text is that most therapists will be interested primarily in treatment evaluation. The arena of treatment evaluation is where single system strategies will have their widest application and greatest impact. Single system procedures can become an integral part of clinical practice when treatment evaluation is the goal. Information related to the scientific legitimacy of the treatment procedures will also be gathered as a by-product of this process.

Practitioners should be careful to never do formal treatment research in the name of treatment evaluation. If a therapist selects a treatment or an outcome measure primarily to answer a question about the treatment or outcome measure per se and not because of a client's need, the activity should be classified as treatment research, not treatment evaluation. If a therapist selects a client for treatment to help answer a predetermined question or investigate a hypothesis of interest, this is treatment research, not treatment evaluation. If the therapist provides a new, costly, time-consuming treatment or measure not directly related to client improvement but designed to strengthen a data base, this is treatment research, not treatment evaluation. In all of the above cases in which single system strategies are being used as methods of treatment research, the clients must be considered research subjects and afforded all the appropriate protections (Barlow et al., 1984).

Single system designs, as argued in previous chapters, can be used to address several important issues related to treatment evaluation with individual clients. The most basic issue is documenting whether a particular treatment is responsible for change in client performance. This issue can be addressed by use of any one of the several single system designs presented previously. In addition, certain designs allow comparison of alternative treatments or of combinations of treatments for a given client. In treatment evaluation, the therapist is primarily concerned with trying to produce change and make decisions about modifying treatments in light of the client's progress. Single system designs permit changes to be made in the course of ongoing treatment and evaluation of client progress.

The practicing therapist is not always interested in the full gamut of scientific questions related to treatment research. Although these questions are of scientific importance, to examine them with single system strategies may not be appropriate or even possible. The practicing clinician is most often interested in basic outcome questions, such as whether an intervention produces change, whether one treatment works better than another for a specific client, or whether a combination of alternative treatments is superior to the constituent treatments alone. All of these questions can be answered within the context of treatment evaluation in which the emphasis is on the improvement of client function.

Thus, the single system strategies described in this book can be used in a variety of contexts. For the majority of therapists, the most useful context will be as techniques in treatment evaluation primarily to systematically document client change and secondarily to contribute empirical information related to developing a scientifically respected clinical practice. The procedures can also be used in other contexts, such as treatment research. Therapists must be astute in their application of the single system strategies presented in this text and bear in mind the ethical implications related to their use.

_____ CONCLUDING REMARKS _____

Single system strategies provide a valuable methodology that can be incorporated into clinical practice at various levels. Key requirements for the use of the designs are monitoring of client progress over time and comparison of client performance before and during intervention. These features are implicit in clinical practice. The goodness of fit between informed clinical decision making and single system procedures is very high. Good clinical practice can be considered synonymous with treatment evaluation in which single system strategies are employed, in that the logic of the two enterprises is so similar. Therapists engaged in good practice are already conducting evaluations of potential scientific value with most of the clients they treat. These therapists need only (1) to take systematic repeated measurements, (2) to specify their treatments, (3) to recognize the design strategies that they are already using, and (4) to use existing design elements deliberately to improve clinical decision making.

Sometimes, it is assumed that occupational and physical therapists are not interested in evaluating or researching the effectiveness of their treatments (Basmajian, 1975). The lack of rigorous published empirical assessments of many treatment procedures as they are practiced in the clinic does not necessarily support this assumption. In fact, a systematic methodology has not been generally available to therapists for evaluating applications of treatment with the individual client. As noted previously, the use of group-comparison research procedures requiring the accumulation of homogeneous samples to which standard treatments can be applied is simply not feasible in general clinical practice. For clinical evaluation to be possible, a methodology is required that is compatible with the characteristics, demands, and priorities of clinical environments. Single system strategies provide such a methodology. Single system designs define the evaluation and treatment process and systematize the manner in which intervention results are incorporated into clinical practice. Systematically evaluating client performance over time and applying treatment according to a design criteria strengthens the inferences that can be drawn regarding treatment efficacy.

Single system evaluation strategies are not a panacea. They cannot, by themselves, ''improve'' the quality of a client's function. They represent a tool which can be of use to therapists in demonstrating to others, and to themselves, that their intervention procedures do make a difference. In the final analysis, proper use and interpretation of single system strategies depends on a complete understanding of the evaluation process, which includes the need for systematic documentation as well as the logic associated with applied approaches to clinical investigation. The basic principles inherent in the application of single system procedures, which includes the need for repeated or continuous collection of data, the manipulation of treatment, the importance of baseline measures, and the interpretation of client response patterns, are far more critical than the knowledge of any particular design. It is hoped that the designs and procedures presented in this book will not be applied in a simple cookbook fashion. It is true, however, that when working in the ''kitchen'' there is often more need for a cookbook than for a textbook describing food chemistry or the biological basis of nutrition. The preceding chapters provide therapists with both the recipes and rationale needed to function effectively in the clinical ''kitchen.''

Therapists should consider the material presented in this book as illustrative and avoid drawing final conclusions concerning any of the procedures presented. The information contained in this text should serve as a basic framework for the development of creative, new, single system procedures applicable to occupational and physical therapy clinical practice. In the final analysis, there are no unalterable recipes for conducting evaluations of therapeutic outcomes. Innumerable permutations, modifications, and combinations of single system strategies are possible, and these new procedures will help solve problems that arise as therapists apply single system strategies in occupational and physical therapy practice.

Glossary

AB design. A single system design that involves two phases: A, in which the baseline data are collected before treatment is implemented, and B, in which data are recorded while treatment is underway.

ABA design. A basic single system design in which the dependent variable is continuously measured across a baseline or pretreatment phase (A), a phase in which intervention is introduced (B), and a second A phase in which intervention is terminated. The ABA design is considered a "stronger" design than the simple AB design because it provides a second A phase during which the client's behaviors or performance can be evaluated once treatment has been withdrawn.

ABAB design. A single system design that involves four phases. The first A represents baseline before treatment is implemented. The first B represents initial application of treatment. The second A designates removal of treatment and a return to baseline conditions. The second B represents a return to treatment conditions. The design is sometimes referred to as a reversal or withdrawal design.

Alternating treatment design. A single system design in which one or more interventions are alternated and/or counterbalanced session by session (or within sessions) rather than over time. Alternations in the treatments may occur over brief periods, in contrast to multiple baseline and ABAB designs in which a degree of stability is needed in the data before a new condition is introduced. This design is also referred to as multielement or multischedule design.

Autocorrelation. The correlation that is present in a set of data collected from an individual or group over time. The data are gathered repeatedly from the same source, and the data points are, therefore, not independent. The degree of autocorrelation or serial dependency in a data set reflects the degree to which a given observation can be predicted by any other observation in the data series.

BAB design. A variation of the basic AB design in which the treatment is introduced in the first phase (B), withdrawn in the second phase (A), and then reintroduced in the third phase (B). The appeal of this design is that it does not require an initial baseline period in which the client receives no intervention.

Bar graph. See *Histogram*.

Baseline. The phase or phases of a single system design in which data are recorded on the untreated client. Frequently, this is the first phase of the design in which data are recorded before treatment is initiated. Performance under this condition is compared with performance during the treatment phase or phases.

Behavior. Any measurable or observable movement, task, or activity of a client. The behavior may be covert (occurring within the individual) or overt. The focus is on measurability and countability; an activity must be definable, observable, or countable in some manner to be considered a behavior.

Carryover effect. Any temporary or permanent change in a client's behavior or performance due to prior exposure to one or more treatment procedures that may contaminate or otherwise influence the client's performance in subsequent periods of treatment.

Case study. The collection of data, both formal and anecdotal, on a single individual or single social unit (e.g., family), with all available evidence from records, observations, and interviews used. In the typical case study, there is no attempt to formally manipulate an independent variable or to identify a dependent variable.

Ceiling effect. An effect that occurs when the performance range of a task or test is so restricted or limited at the upper end that the clients cannot perform to their maximum ability.

Celeration line. A line of progress computed from a data series. The celeration line represents a line of best fit that divides the data points into equal halves and visually indicates the trend of the data series. Celeration is derived from the direction that the trend may be progressing, i.e., accelerating or decelerating.

Changing criterion design. A single system design in which the expectation for performance or behavior changes for each phase of the design. The design is particularly useful for behaviors that demonstrate stepwise sequential improvement.

Control group. A group of subjects selected in a way that makes them comparable with participants in the treatment group, except that, unlike those in the treatment group, they are not exposed to the independent variable.

Correlation. Generally, the type of statistical analysis used in studies of a relation between variables. Correlational studies investigate the degree to which two or more variables, such as height and weight, vary together in a population.

Counterbalancing. Any systematic procedure designed to distribute various carryover effects so that they will not interfere with the effect produced by the treatment.

Criterion variable. See *Dependent variable.*

Cumulative graph. A graphic presentation of successive combined numbers or scores (rate, frequency, percent, duration) representative of client performance or behavior.

Data. Generally, the information gathered during the course of an evaluation to answer the question being investigated. The term *data* covers all information that may be recorded for a client, such as age, sex, or performance scores, and usually is used with reference to the dependent variable.

Data point. Any point on a graph that represents the value for the dependent variable for an individual or group of observations. Although the term *data* may refer to any part or all of a set of information, the term *data point* implies the visual representation of that information.

Data transformation. Any procedure that changes all the values in a data series by the same function. Data transformations are typically employed to simplify computations, to obtain scores having a standardized distribution, and to obtain a dependent variable that meets assumptions required for statistical analysis.

Dependent variable. That variable being measured in a study or evaluation. If, for example, the goal of treatment was to increase upper extremity range of motion, the dependent variable would be the range of motion displayed by the client. The dependent variable is also referred to as the criterion variable or outcome measure.

Duration recording. The recording of the duration or time that a behavior or performance event lasts.

Ecological validity. A form of external validity that refers to whether the results of an evaluation or an investigation can be generalized to other settings beyond the setting in which the evaluation occurred.

Empirical (empiricism). An approach to inquiry which emphasizes knowledge that comes through factual investigation, with the facts obtained from sources external to the evaluator or investigator. Direct experience or objective observation and measurement are the primary means by which information is obtained.

Evaluation. The analysis or comparison of data, collected during a measurement period in a systematic defined manner, on which decisions concerning client treatment can be based. The primary emphasis during evaluation is on client improvement and decision making in relation to client needs.

Ex post facto **design.**   Any research design in which subjects are classified on the basis of whether or not, or to what degree, they were
exposed to some naturally occurring event rather than to an event
manipulated or controlled by the investigator.

Experimental group.   See *Treatment group.*

Experimental mortality.   A threat to internal validity which occurs when
a loss of subjects changes the composition of a sample. When this
occurs, particularly if more subjects are lost from one group than from
another group, the investigator may not have groups that are con-
stituted in the same way that they were when the study was initiated.

External validity.   The generalizability of results from a given investigation or evaluation. External validity refers to how well the results
of a particular investigation apply to the world outside the evaluation
situation. If an evaluation is externally valid, one can expect that the
results are generalizable to other settings and individuals.

Floor (Basal) effect.   An effect that occurs when the performance range
of a task or test is so restricted or limited on the lower end that the
client's performance is determined by the task or test rather than by
their ability to perform. Under such conditions, the task or test is so
difficult that the investigator is unable to obtain any evidence about
how the clients can perform.

Frequency recording.   A tally or frequency count of discrete events or
client performance as it occurs. This is also referred to as event
recording.

Group design.   Any design in which data are collected from an assem-
blage of subjects rather than from subjects one at a time. This also
refers to any design in which groups are the experimental unit of
interest and the dependent variable is a group score.

Histogram (bar graph).   A format for illustrating data. The rectangular
columns (bars) represent values of the x-axis; the height of each bar
indicates the amount of the dependent variable (y-axis) associated with
each value on the x-axis.

History.   A threat to internal validity that occurs when specific events, in
addition to the treatment, intervene between measurements and affect
the outcome or performance on the dependent variable.

Hypothesis.   A statement used in research to help clarify the research
question. It is presented as a declarative statement of prediction. Two
basic formats are used, the *null* hypothesis and the *directional* hypothesis. The null hypothesis usually predicts no difference, while the
directional hypothesis predicts a difference and the direction of that
difference.

Idiographic.   Pertains to or emphasizes the individual case or event. In single system strategies, idiographic refers to any system for the assessment of behavior or performance derived from a particular individual rather than from the average of many individuals' performance.

Independent variable. That variable or phenomenon that is under investigation or that factor that the investigator manipulates to see what effect is produced. For example, if the evaluator wanted to determine whether a series of exercises could reduce low back pain, the series of exercises would be the independent variable (treatment) and low back pain would be the dependent variable.

Instrumentation. A threat to internal validity that occurs when changes in the calibration of a measuring instrument result in alteration of the scores that are recorded. Instrumentation also refers to changes in "calibration" in human observers which may result as a function of systematic differences in the way that the observers judge and record observations.

Interaction design. A complex single system design in which more than one treatment is alternated singly or in combination with other treatments over a series of preplanned phases. The purpose of the design is to determine the additive, subtractive, and interactive effect of a given treatment alone or in combination with other treatments.

Internal validity. The technical soundness of a study. An investigation is internally valid or has high internal validity when all the potential factors that might influence performance on the outcome measure are controlled, except the one under study. When an investigation has high internal validity, the investigator can be confident that the independent variable (treatment) was responsible for any change found on the dependent variable.

Interobserver agreement measures. Procedures to verify the reliability of the measurement of client performance or behavior. Reliability is usually concerned with the percentage of agreement among two or more independent observers or the occurrence or nonoccurrence of a behavior or performance event.

Intervention. See *Treatment*.

Level. The magnitude of the data as indicated by the value on the y-axis. Changes in level are associated with abrupt changes in performance that occur when one phase ends and the next phase begins. A change in level from one phase to the next is called a discontinuity in the data series.

Maturation. A threat to internal validity that occurs when factors influence performance as a result of time passing. Such factors as growing older, physical development, and emotional development are considered maturational threats to internal validity when they influence performance on the outcome measure and are not controlled for by the design.

Mean. A descriptive statistic obtained by adding the scores of all clients or the repeated scores for a single client and dividing this sum by the total number of scores. This is also referred to as the arithmetic average.

Measurement. The systematic and objective quantification of objects, events, or behaviors according to a predetermined set of rules. Basic steps in measurement are (1) to identify what is to be measured, (2) to define what is to be measured in operational, observable terms, and (3) to select an appropriate data-recording system for recording behavior or performance events.

Multiple baseline design. A single system design in which data are collected for more than one subject, behavior, or setting. Phase changes from baseline to intervention across subjects, behaviors, or settings are staggered so that sequential control for the subject, behavior, or setting prior to treatment is demonstrated.

Multiple probe design. A variation of the multiple baseline design. In the multiple probe design, the independent variable is systematically and sequentially introduced to one subject (or in one setting, or with one behavior) at a time. Data are collected, however, during probe trials rather than on a continuous basis, as occurs in the multiple baseline design.

Nomothetic. Pertains to general principles and laws. In behavioral science research, nomothetic refers to any system for the assessment of behavior or performance which is based on the average of many individuals' performance.

Nonconcurrent multiple baseline. A version of the multiple baseline design across subjects. In this design, the baseline periods are predetermined and the baseline lengths are randomly assigned to clients as they become available for evaluation. The baseline periods are not begun concurrently for all the clients involved in the evaluation.

Nonreactive measure. A measure of behavior or performance which minimizes the client's awareness of being evaluated and thus reduces the tendency to react in ways that produce artifacts or other distortions of the data.

Operational definition. A process whereby the investigator specifies all the steps (operations) and details associated with the dependent and the independent variable included in an evaluation. In the operational definition of variables, each term is taken in turn, and exactly what is meant by that term is specified.

Order effects.   A sequencing effect that arises from the order in which the treatment conditions are administered.

Percent correct performance.   The number of times that a behavior occurs correctly per total number of opportunities for the behavior to occur, multiplied by 100; i.e., the number "correct" divided by the number of opportunities and multiplied by 100 equals the percentage of correct responses.

Phase change.   That moment when conditions are changed in single system designs. There may be several phase changes, such as the moment when the baseline condition is terminated and the treatment is begun, or the moment when treatment is terminated and the baseline or untreated condition is reinstituted (as in an ABAB design).

Population validity.   A form of external validity that refers to whether the results of an evaluation or investigation can be generalized to other individuals who are members of the target population.

Population.   Any well-described set of people or events from which the investigator selects a sample of subjects or clients.

Practical significance.   A change in client behavior or performance that is regarded as personally and socially significant by an individual client and those in contact with the client.

Pretest/posttest control group design.   A research design in which one or more groups of randomly assigned subjects are observed or measured before and after a treatment is introduced. The control group is measured in the same way, and scores are then compared. These comparisons may be among posttest scores only, or they may be among difference scores obtained by subtracting a subject's pretest score from his or her posttest score.

Pure (basic) research.   Research conducted with the primary intent of increasing general information or scientific knowledge, without regard to immediate practical application of the information.

Quasi-experimental design.   A research design in which subjects frequently are not randomly assigned to conditions, although the independent variable may be manipulated. Subjects are not randomly assigned to conditions usually because it is impossible or not feasible to do so.

Random assignment.   A procedure for determining the assignment of subjects to conditions in such a way that the probability of being assigned to a particular condition is the same for all subjects participating in the investigation.

Random sampling.   A selection procedure whereby each individual in the population has an equal chance of being chosen as a participant in the investigation. This is also known as simple random sampling.

Rate recording.   The frequency of occurrence of a behavior or performance event as a unit of time. Rate is calculated by dividing the frequency of occurrence by a unit of time; i.e., rate = frequency/time, and is often expressed in responses per minute.

Raw data.   Data first recorded during the evaluation or investigation, prior to the performance of operations that reduce, consolidate, or transform them.

Reactivity.   Changes in the client or the environment that result in the outcome measure due to the act of recording or measurement and not due to the treatment.

Research.   A systematic way of asking questions and discovering information that relies on an orderly method of inquiry known as the scientific method.

Sample.   Those individuals or events that are selected from the population to serve as the participants in a study or investigation. This term is also used as a verb (to sample) and, as a verb, refers to the process of selecting individuals to serve as participants in an investigation.

Serial dependence.   See *Autocorrelation*.

Simple line graph.   Sometimes referred to as a noncumulative graph. Client scores are placed on squared graph paper. The amount of behavior (y-axis) is plotted at the intersection of the time section (x-axis). After scores (data points) have been placed on the graph, they are connected by a line to form a data path.

Simultaneous treatment design.   A single system design that requires the simultaneous or concurrent application of two or more interventions with a single client (or small group). In the simultaneous treatment design, all interventions are presented or available to the client at the same time. This is also referred to as the concurrent schedule design.

Single system design.   A design based on idiographic principles that requires the repeated collection of information on a single system over time with use of well-defined systematic procedures. This is also referred to as single-subject research, single-case experimental designs, time-series designs, intrasubject designs, or idiographic designs.

Slope.   The rate of change described by a line. The slope of a line is equal to the vertical difference between any two points on the line divided by the horizontal difference between the same two points.

Social validity.   Refers to whether the focus of the intervention (goals) and the behavior or performance change achieved by the individual meet the demands of the social community and milieu of which the client is a part.

Stability. See *Variability*.

Standard deviation. A descriptive statistic that is the most commonly used index of variability. The standard deviation may be conceptualized as a measure of the variability in scores around the mean.

Statistical regression. A threat to internal validity which occurs when subjects have been assigned to a group or condition on the basis of extreme or atypical scores. When the subject is tested a second time, his or her score may show a natural regression to the mean, which may erroneously be interpreted as due to a treatment effect.

Statistical significance testing. The use of a statistical test to provide a probability statement when a decision is made regarding the tenability of the null hypothesis of no relationship between two or more variables.

Statistical significance. The value that is arbitrarily selected usually $p <$ .05, to define the test statistic (e.g., t or F test) as too large to make the null hypothesis tenable.

Testing. A threat to internal validity that occurs when the effect of taking a test substantially influences the scores of participants on a second testing.

Time sampling. The measurement of the occurrence or the non-occurrence of a behavior or performance event immediately following a specified interval of time.

Treatment. A systematically formulated set of principles and procedures that are used to modify and improve client performance or behavior.

Treatment evaluation. The use of systematic and objective procedures to assess the progress or improvement of a client receiving therapy services. The primary emphasis is on collecting information that will enhance client function. A secondary goal is to gather information designed to answer questions of scientific interest and to generate an empirical knowledge base for a particular treatment or theory.

Treatment group. The group(s) assigned to receive the independent variable or treatment. The effect of the independent variable is assessed by comparison among treatment groups or between treatment and control groups.

Treatment research. The use of systematic and objective procedures designed to answer questions of scientific interest, to generate scientifically valid statements, or to test hypotheses related to a specific independent variable. A secondary goal is to benefit the individuals who participate in the research investigation. The individual client needs are accommodated within the framework and requirements of the research investigation.

Trend. Directionality in a data series. The data series may be increasing, decreasing, or stationary. If the data points in the data series are generally moving in a linear upward direction, an accelerating trend is suggested. Trends can occur both within a phase and across phases.

Variability. The amount of fluctuation or instability in a data series. A data series with considerable variability will be depicted graphically by a data path with numerous peaks and valleys.

Variable. Any condition or factor in the individual or environment, whether manipulated or observed, which changes or can be changed during the course of an investigation. See also *Dependent variable* and *Independent variable*.

Visual inspection. The process of reaching a judgment about the reliability or consistency of intervention effects by visually examining the graphed data.

X-axis. The x-axis is the horizontal axis (abscissa) in a standard equal interval graphic arrangement and usually indicates units of time (e.g., minutes, hours, days, weeks) or trials.

Y-axis. The y-axis is the vertical axis (ordinate) in a standard equal interval graphic arrangement and usually indicates the amount of behavior or performance (e.g., frequency, rate, percentage, duration).

References

Altman, J. (1974). Observational study of behavior: Sampling methods. *Behavior, 49,* 227–267.

Anderson, S. C., and Ball, S. (1978). *The profession and practice of program evaluation.* San Francisco: Jossey-Bass.

Baer, D. M. (1977). Perhaps it would be better not to know everything. *J. Appl. Behav. Anal., 10,* 167–172.

Bakan, D. (1966). The test of significance in psychological research. *Psychol. Bull., 66,* 423–437.

Ballin, A. J., Breslin, W. H., Wierenga, K. A., and Shepard, K. F. (1980). Research in physical therapy: Philosophy, barriers to involvement, and use among California physical therapists. *Phys. Ther., 60,* 888–895.

Barlow, D., Hayes, S. C., and Nelson, R. O. (1984). *The scientist practitioner. Research and accountability in clinical and educational settings.* New York: Pergamon Press.

Barlow, D. H., and Hayes, S. C. (1979). Alternating treatment design: One strategy for comparing the effects of two treatments in a single subject. *J. Appl. Behav. Anal., 3,* 73–76.

Barlow, D. H., and Hersen, M. (1973). Single-case experimental designs. *Arch. Gen. Psychiatry, 29,* 319–325.

Barlow, D. H., and Hersen, M. (1984). *Single case experimental designs: Strategies for studying behavior change* (2nd ed.) New York: Pergamon Press.

Basmajian, J. V. (1975). Research or retrench: The rehabilitation fields challenged. *Phys. Ther., 55,* 607–610.

Basmajian, J. V. (1977). Professional survival: The role of research in physical therapy. *Phys. Ther., 57,* 283–285.

Bayley, N. (1969). *Bayley scales of infant development.* New York: Psychological Corp.

Bijou, S. W. (1966). A functional analysis of retarded behavior. In N. R. Ellis (Ed.), *International review of research in mental retardation* (Vol. 1). New York: Academic Press.

Bijou, S. W., Peterson, R. F., and Ault, M. H. (1968). A method to integrate descriptive and experimental field studies at the level of data and empirical concepts. *J. Appl. Behav. Anal., 1,* 175–191.

Birnbauer, J. S. (1981). External validity and experimental investigation of individual behavior. *Anal. Intervent. Dev. Disabil., 1,* 117–132.

Bloom, M. (1975). *The paradox of helping: Introduction to the philosophy of scientific practice.* New York: Macmillan Publishing.

Bloom, M., and Fischer, J. (1982). *Evaluating practice: Guidelines for the accountable professional.* Englewood Cliffs, NJ: Prentice-Hall.

Blumberg, C. J. (1984). Comments on a "A simplified time-series analysis for evaluating treatment interventions." *J. Appl. Behav. Anal., 17,* 539–542.

Bolgar, H. (1965). The case study method. In B. B. Wolman (Ed.), *Handbook of clinical psychology.* New York: McGraw-Hill.

Bonadonna, P. (1981). Effects of vestibular stimulation program on sterotypic rocking behavior. *Am. J. Occup. Ther., 35,* 775–782.

Bracht, G. H., and Glass, G. V. (1968). The external validity of experiments. *Am. Educ. Res. J., 5,* 437–474.

Burr, W. R., Mead, P. E., and Rollins, B. C. (1973). A model for the application of research findings by the educator and counselor: Research to theory to practice. *Fam. Coordinator, 23,* 285–290.

Campbell, D. T. (1969). Prospective: Artifact and control. In R. Rosenthal and R. L. Rosnow (Eds.), *Artifacts in behavioral research.* New York: Academic Press.

Campbell D. T., and Stanley, J. C. (1963). Experimental and quasi-experimental design for research. In N. L. Gage (Ed.), *Handbook of research on teaching.* Chicago: Rand McNally.

Carr, B. S., and Williams, M. (1982). Analysis of therapeutic techniques through the use of the Standard Behavior Chart. *Phys. Ther., 62,* 177–183.

Cartwright, C. A., and Cartwright, G. P. (1974). *Developing observational skills.* New York: McGraw-Hill.

Carver, R. P. (1978). The case against statistical significance testing. *Harvard Educ. Rev., 48,* 378–399.

Chassan, J. B. (1979). *Research design in clinical psychology and psychiatry* (2nd ed.). New York: Irvington Press.

Chee, F., Kreutzberg, J., and Clark, D. (1978). Semicircular canal stimulation in cerebral palsied children. *Phys. Ther., 58,* 1071–1075.

Christensen, L. B. (1980). *Experimental methodology* (2nd ed.). Boston: Allyn & Bacon.

Christiansen, C. H. (1981). Editorial: Toward resolution of crisis: Research requisites in occupational therapy. *Occup. Ther. J. Res., 1,* 115–124.

Christiansen, C. H. (1983). Editorial-research: An economic imperative. *Occup. Ther. J. Res., 3,* 195–198.

Connolly, B., Craik, R., and Krebs, D. E. (1983). Single-case research: When is it valid? Guest editorial. *Phys. Ther., 63,* 1767–1768.

Cook, T. D., and Campbell, D. T. (1979). *Quasi-experimentation design & analysis issues for field settings.* Boston: Houghton-Mifflin.

Cook, T. D., and Reichardt, C. S. (Eds.) (1979). *Qualitative and quantitative methods in evaluation research.* Beverly Hills: Sage Publications.

Cooper, H. M. (1981a). On the significance of effects and the effects of significance. *J. Pers. Soc. Psychol., 41,* 1013–1018.

Cooper, J. V. (1981b). *Measuring behavior* (2nd ed.). Columbus, OH: Charles E. Merrill.

Cox, R. S., and West, W. (1982). *Fundamentals of research for health professionals.* Laurel, MD: RAMSCO.

Cronbach, L. J. (1982). *Designing evaluations of education and social programs.* San Francisco: Jossey-Bass.

Cubie, S. H., and Kaplan, K. (1982). A case analysis method for the model of human occupation. *Am. J. Occup. Ther., 36,* 645–657.

Cuvo, A. J. (1979). Multiple-baseline designs in instructional research: Pitfalls of measurement and procedural advantages. *Am. J. Ment. Defic., 89,* 219–228.

DeProspero, A., and Cohen, S. C. (1979). Inconsistent visual analysis of intrasubject data. *J. Appl. Behav. Anal., 12,* 573–579.

Denenberg, V. H. (1978). Paradigms and paradoxes in the study of behavioral development. In E. B. Thoman (Ed.), *The origins of the infant's social responsiveness*. Hillsdale, NJ: Lawrence Erlbaum.

Dubois, E. N. (1964). *Essential methods in business statistics*. New York: McGraw-Hill.

Edington, E. S. (1980). Validity of randomization tests for one-subject experiments. *J. Educ. Stat., 5*, 235–251.

Edington, E. S. (1982). Nonparametric tests for single-subject multiple schedule experiments. *Behav. Assessment, 4*, 83–91.

Edwards, A. L. (1967). *Statistical methods* (2nd ed.). New York: Holt, Rinehart & Winston.

Elashoff, J. D., and Thoresen , C. E. (1978). Choosing a statistical method for analysis of an intensive experiment. In T. R. Kratochwill (Ed.), *Single subject research: Strategies for evaluating change*. New York: Academic Press.

Epstein, S. (1980). The stability of behavior: Implications for psychological research. *Am. Psychol., 35*, 790–806.

Fisher, R. A. (1925). *Statistical methods for research workers*. Edinburgh: Oliver & Boyd.

Fishman, S. T. (1981). Narrowing the generalization gap in clinical research. *Behav. Assessment, 3*, 243–248.

Fuhrer, M. J. (1983). Communicating and utilizing research in medical rehabilitation. *Arch. Phys. Med. Rehabil., 64*, 608–610.

Furlong, M. J., and Wampold, B. (1981). Visual analysis of single-subject studies by school psychologists. *Psychol. Schools, 18*, 80–86.

Furlong, M. J., and Wampold, B. (1982). Intervention effects and relative variation as dimensions in experts' use of visual inference. *J. Appl. Behav. Anal., 15*, 415–421.

Gentile, J. R., Roden, A. H., and Klein, R. D. (1972). An analysis of variance model for the intrasubject replication design. *J. Appl. Behav. Anal., 5*, 193–198.

Gilbert, J. P., Light, R. S., and Mosteller, F. (1975). Assessing social innovations: An empirical basis for policy. In C. A. Bennett and A. A. Lumsdaine (Eds.), *Evaluation and experiment*. New York: Academic Press.

Gillette, N. P. (1982). Nationally speaking—A data base for occupational therapy. *Am. J. Occup. Ther., 36*, 499–501.

Glass, G. V., Wilson, V. L., and Gottman, J. M. (1975). *Design and analysis of time series experiments*. Boulder: Colorado Associated University Press.

Goode, W. (1969). The theoretical limits of professionalism. In A. Etzion (Ed.), *The semi-professions and their organization*. New York: Free Press.

Goodisman, L. D. (1982). A manipulation-free design for single-subject cerebral palsy research. *Phys. Ther., 62*, 284–289.

Gortner, S. R., and Nahm, H. (1977). An overview of nursing research in the United States. *Nurs. Res., 26*, 10–23.

Gortner, S. R. (1975). Research for a practice profession. *Nurs. Res., 24*, 193–197.

Gottman, J. M., and Glass, G. V. (1978). Analysis of interrupted time-series experiments. In T. R. Kratochwill (Ed.), *Single-subject research: Strategies for evaluating change*. New York: Academic Press.

Gottman, J. M., and Leiblum, S. R. (1974). *How to do psychotherapy and how to evaluate it*. New York: Holt, Rinehart & Winston.

Greenwald, A. (1975). Consequences of prejudice against the null hypothesis. *Psychol. Bull., 82*, 1–20.

Hacker, B. (1980). Single subject research strategies in occupational therapy. Part 1. *Am. J. Occup. Ther., 34*, 103–108.

Harris, F. C., and Lahey, B. B. (1978). A method for combining occurrence and non-occurrence interobserver agreement scores. *J. Appl. Behav. Anal., 11*, 523–527.

Hartmann, D. P. (1974). Forcing square pegs into round holes: Some comments on "An analysis-of-variance model for the intersubject replication design." *J. Appl. Behav. Anal., 7,* 635–638.

Hartmann, D. P., Gottman, J. M., Jones, R. R., Gardner, W., Kazdin, A. E., and Vaught, R. (1980). Interrupted time-series analysis and its application to behavioral data. *J. Appl. Behav. Anal., 10,* 103–116.

Hawkins, R. P. (1979). The function of assessment: Implications for selection and development of devices for assessing repertories in clinical, and other settings. *J. Appl. Behav. Anal., 21,* 501–516.

Hawkins, R. P. (1982). Developing a behavior code. In D. P. Hartmann (Ed.), *Using observations to study behavior: New directions for methodology of social and behavioral science* (pp. 21–35). San Francisco: Jossey-Bass.

Hawkins, R. P., Axelrod, S., and Hall, R. V. (1976). Teachers as behavior analysts: Precisely monitoring student performance. In J. A. Brigham, R. P. Hawkins, J. Scott, and J. F. McLaughlin (Eds.), *Behavior analysis in education: Self-control and reading.* Dubuque, IA: Kendall-Hunt.

Hawkins, R. P., and Dotson, V. A. (1975). Reliability scores that delude: An Alice in Wonderland trip through the misleading characteristics of interobserver agreement scores in interval recording. In E. Ramp and G. Semb (Eds.), *Behavior analysis: Areas of research and application.* Englewood Cliffs, NJ: Prentice-Hall.

Hayes, S. C. (1981). Single case experimental design and empirical clinical practice. *J. Consult. Clin. Psychol., 49,* 193–211.

Haynes, S. N. (1978). *Principles of behavioral assessment.* New York: Gardner Press.

Haynes, S. N., and Horn, W. F. (1982). Reactivity in behavioral observation: A review. *Behav. Assessment, 4,* 369–385.

Hemphill, J. K. (1969). The relationship between research and evaluation studies. In R. W. Tyler (Ed.), *Educational evaluation: New roles, new means* (pp. 242–283), Chicago: NSSE.

Herbert, J., and Attridge, C. (1975). A guide for developers and users of observation systems and manuals. *Am. Educ. Res. J., 12,* 1–20.

Hersen, M. (1973). Self assessment of fear. *Behav. Ther., 4,* 241–257.

Hersen, M., and Barlow, D. H. (1976). *Single-case experimental design: Strategies for behavior change.* New York: Pergamon Press.

Hislop, H. J. (1975). The not-so-impossible dream. *Phys. Ther., 55,* 1069–1080.

Horner, R. D., and Baer, D. M. (1978). Multiple-probe technique: A variation of the multiple baseline. *J. Appl. Behav. Anal., 11,* 189–196.

Huitema, B. (1985). Autocorrelation in applied behavior analysis: A myth. *Behav. Assess., 7,* 107–113.

Huitema, B., and Girman, S. (1978). *The statistical structure of behavior modification data.* Paper presented at the fourth annual Midwest Association of Behavior Analysis convention, Chicago.

Hunt, J. (1981). Indicators for nursing practice: The use of research findings. *J. Advanced Nurs., 6,* 189–194.

Isaac, S., and Michael, W. B. (1971). *Handbook in research and evaluation.* San Diego: EDITS.

Jackson, D. A., and Wallace, R. F. (1974). The modification and generalization of voice loudness in a fifteen-year-old retarded girl. *J. Appl. Behav. Anal., 7,* 461–471.

Jayaratne, S., and Levy, R. L. (1979). *Empirical clinical practice.* New York: Columbia University Press.

Johnson, S. M., and Bolstad, O. D. (1973). Methodological issues in naturalistic observation: Some problems and solutions for field research. In L. A. Hamerlynck, L. C.

Handy and E. I. Mash (Eds.), *Behavior change: Methodology, concepts and practice.* Champaign, IL: Research Press.

Johnston, J. M., and Pennypacker, H. S. (1980). *Strategies and tactics of human behavioral research.* Hillsdale, NJ: Lawrence Erlbaum.

Jones, R. R., Crowell, D. H., and Kapunia, L. E. (1969). Change detection model for serially correlated data. *Psych. Bull., 71*, 352–358.

Jones, R. R., Vaught, R. S., and Weinrott, M. R. (1977). Time-series analysis in operant research. *J. Appl. Behav. Anal., 10*, 151–156.

Jones, R. R., Weinrott, M. R., and Vaught, R. S. (1978). Effects of serial dependency on the agreement between visual and statistical inferences. *J. Appl. Behav. Anal., 11*, 277–283.

Kauffman, J. M., and Hallahan, D. P. (1974). The medical model and the science of special education. *Except. Child., 41*, 97–102.

Kazdin, A. E. (1976). Statistical analysis for single-case experimental designs. In M. Hersen and D. H. Barlow (Eds.) *Single-case experimental designs: Strategies for studying behavior change.* New York: Pergamon Press.

Kazdin, A. E. (1977). Assessing the clinical or applied significance of behavior change through social validation. *Behav. Modification, 1*, 427–452.

Kazdin, A. E. (1978). Methodological and interpretive problems of single case experimental designs. *J. Consult. Clin. Psychol., 46*, 629–642.

Kazdin, A. E. (1979). Unobtrusive measures in behavioral assessment. *J. Appl. Behav. Anal., 12*, 713–724.

Kazdin, A. E. (1980). *Research design in clinical psychology.* New York: Harper & Row.

Kazdin, A. E. (1982). *Single-case research designs: Methods for clinical and applied settings.* New York: Oxford University Press.

Kazdin, A. E. (1983). Single-case research in clinical child psychiatry. *J. Am. Acad. Child Psychiatry, 22*, 423–432.

Kazdin, A. E., and Hartmann, D. P. (1978). The simultaneous treatment design. *Behav. Ther., 9*, 912–922.

Kelly, M. B. (1977). A review of the observational data-collection and reliability procedures reported in the *Journal of Applied Behavioral Analysis. J. Appl. Behav. Anal., 10*, 97–101.

Keppel, G. (1973). *Design and analysis: A researcher's handbook.* Englewood Cliffs, NJ: Prentice-Hall.

Kerlinger, F. N. (1973). *Foundations of behavioral research* (2nd ed.). New York: Holt, Rinehart & Winston.

Kerlinger, F. N. (1979). *Behavioral research: A conceptual approach.* New York: Holt, Rinehart & Winston.

Ketefian, S. (1975). Applications of selected nursing research findings into nursing practice: A pilot study. *Nurs. Res., 24*, 89–92.

Kirk, R. E. (1968). *Experimental design: Procedures for the behavioral sciences.* Monterey, CA: Brooks/Cole.

Koorland, M. A., and Martin, M. B. (1975). *Elementary principles and procedures for the Standard Behavior Chart.* Gainesville, FL: Learning Environments.

Kratochwill, T. R. (Ed.) (1978). *Single subject research: Strategies for evaluating change.* New York: Academic Press.

Kratochwill, T. R., and Brody, G. H. (1978). Single subject designs: A perspective on the controversy over employing statistical inference and implications for research and training in behavior modification. *Behav. Modification, 2*, 291–307.

Kratochwill, T. R., and Levin, R. J. (1980). On the applicability of various data analysis procedures to the simultaneous and alternating treatment designs in behavior therapy research. *Behav. Assessment, 2*, 353–360.

Laskas, C. A., Mullen, S. L., Nelson, D. L., and Broyles, M. W. (1985). Enhancement of two motor functions of the lower extremity in a child with spastic quadriplegia. *Phys. Ther., 65,* 11–16.

Leitenberg, H. (1973). The use of single-case methodology in psychotherapy research. *J. Abnorm. Psychol., 82,* 87–101.

Levy, R. L., and Olson, D. G. (1979). The single-subject methodology in clinical practice: An overview. *J. Soc. Serv. Res., 3,* 25–49.

Llorens, L. (1981). A journal of research in occupational therapy: The need, the response. *Occup. Ther. J. Res., 1,* 3–7.

Lucci, J. A. (1980). *Occupational therapy case studies* (2nd ed.). Garden City, NY: Medical Examination Publishing.   ·

Martin, G., and Pear, J. (1978). *Behavior modification: What it is and how to do it.* Englewood Cliffs, NJ: Prentice-Hall.

Mash, E. J., Terdal, L., and Anderson, K. (1976). The response class matrix: A procedure for recording parent-child interactions. In E. J. Mash and L. B. Terdal (Eds.), *Behavior therapy assessment: Diagnosis, design, and evaluation.* New York: Springer.

McCain, L. J., and McCleary, R. (1979). The statistical analysis of the simple interrupted time-series quasi-experiment. In T. D. Cook and D. T. Campbell (Eds.), *Quasi-experimentation: Design and analysis issues for field settings.* Chicago: Rand McNally.

McDowall, D., McCleary, R., Meidinger, E., and Hay, R. A. (1980). *Interrupted time-series analysis.* (In J. L. Sullivan (Ed.), *Quantitative applications in the social sciences series,* Vol. 21.) Beverly Hills, CA: Sage Publications.

McPherson, J. J., Kreimeyer, D., Aalderks, M., and Gallagher, T. (1982). A comparison of dorsal and volar resting hand splints in the reduction of hypertonus. *Am. J. Occup. Ther., 36,* 664–671.

Michael, J. (1974). Statistical inference for individual organism research: Mixed blessing or curse? *J. Appl. Behav. Anal., 7,* 647–653.

Murphy, R., and Bryan, A. J. (1980). Multiple-baseline and multiple-probe designs: Practical alternatives for special education assessment and evaluation. *J. Spec. Educ., 14,* 325–335.

Nelson, R. O. (1981). Realistic dependent measures for clinical use. *J. Consult. Clin. Psychol., 49,* 168–182.

Nelson, R. O., and Hayes, S. C. (1979). Some current dimensions of behavioral assessment. *Behav. Assessment, 1,* 1–11.

Noonan, M. J. (1984). Teaching postural reactions to students with severe cerebral palsy: An evaluation of theory and technique. *J. Assoc. Severely Handicapped, 9,* 111–122.

Ottenbacher, K. (1982). Statistical power and research in occupational therapy. *Occup. Ther. J. Res., 2,* 13–26.

Ottenbacher, K. (1983). Patterns of postrotary nystagmus in three learning disabled children. *Am. J. Occup. Ther., 36,* 657–663.

Ottenbacher, K. (1984a). The significance of power and the power of significance: Recommendations for occupational therapy research. *Occup. Ther. J. Res., 4,* 38–50.

Ottenbacher, K. (1984b). Nomothetic and idiographic strategies for clinical research: In apposition or opposition. *Occup. Ther. J. Res., 4,* 198–212.

Ottenbacher, K., Hicks, J., Roark, A., and Swinea, J. (1983). Oral sensorimotor therapy in the developmentally disabled: A multiple baseline study. *Am. J. Occup. Ther., 37,* 541–548.

Ottenbacher, K., Scoggins, A., and Wayland, J. (1981). The effectiveness of a program of oral sensory-motor therapy with the severely and profoundly developmentally disabled. *Occup. Ther. J. Res., 1,* 147–160.

Ottenbacher, K., and Short, M. A. (1982). Publication trends in occupational therapy. *Occup. Ther. J. Res., 2,* 80–88.

Ottenbacher, K., and York, J. (1984). Strategies for measuring clinical change: Implications for practice and research. *Am. J. Occup. Ther., 38,* 647–659.

Parsonson, B. S., and Baer, D. M. (1978). The analysis and presentation of graphic data. In T. R. Kratochwill (Ed.), *Single-subject research: Strategies for evaluating change.* New York: Academic Press.

Payton, O. P. (1979). *Research the validation of clinical practice.* Philadelphia: F. A. Davis.

Pennypacker, H. S., Koenig, C. H., and Lindsley, O. R. (1972). *Handbook of the Standard Behavior Chart.* Kansas City, MO: Precision Media.

Popham, W. J. (Ed.). (1974). *Evaluation in education: Current applications.* Berkeley, CA: McCutchan.

Ray, S. A., Bundy, A. C., and Nelson D. (1983). Decreased drooling through techniques to facilitate mouth closure. *Am. J. Occup. Ther., 37,* 749–754.

Reid, J. B. (1970). Reliability assessment of observation data: A possible methodological problem. *Child Dev., 41,* 1143–1150.

Repp, A. C., Roberts, D. M., Slack, D. J., Repp, C. F., and Berkler, M. S. (1976). A comparison of frequency, interval and time sampling methods of data collection. *J. Appl. Behav. Anal., 9,* 501–508.

Robinson, P. W. (1976). *Fundamentals of experimental psychology.* Englewood Cliffs, NJ: Prentice-Hall.

Robinson, P. W., and Foster, D. F. (1979). *Experimental psychology: A small-N approach.* New York: Harper & Row.

Rosenthal, R. (1966). *Experimenter effects in behavioral research.* New York: Appleton-Century-Crofts.

Rosenthal, R., and Rosnow, R. L. (1984). *Essentials of behavioral research: Methods and data analysis.* New York: McGraw-Hill.

Rossi, P. H., and Freeman, H. E. (1982). *Evaluation: A systematic approach* (2nd ed.). Beverly Hills, CA: Sage Publications.

Sackett, G. P. (1978). Measurement in observational research. In G. P. Sackett (Ed.), *Observing behavior: Data collection and analysis methods* (Vol. 2). Baltimore: University Park Press.

Sanders, R. M. (1978). *How to plot data.* Lawrence, KS: H & H Enterprises.

Schenkenberg, T., Bradford, D. C., and Ajax, E. (1980). Line bisection and unilateral visual neglect in patients with neurologic impairment. *Neurology, 30,* 509–517.

Sidman, M. (1960). *Tactics of scientific research.* New York: Basic Books.

Siegel, S. (1956). *Nonparametric statistics.* New York: McGraw-Hill.

Smith, D., and Snell, M. E. (1978). Classroom management and instructional planning. In M. E. Snell (Ed.), *Systematic instruction of the moderately and severely handicapped.* Columbus, OH, Charles E. Merrill.

Smith, P. C., and Kendall, L. M. (1963). Retranslation of expectations: An approach to the construction of unambiguous anchors for rating scales. *J. Appl. Psychol., 47,* 149–155.

Sobsey, R., and Orelove, F. P. (1984). Neurophysiological facilitation of eating skills in children with severe handicaps. *J. Assoc. Severely Handicapped, 9,* 98–110.

Stake, R. E., and Denny, T. (1969). Needed concepts and techniques for utilizing more fully the potential of evaluation. In R. W. Tyler (Ed.), *Educational evaluation: New roles, new means* (pp. 370–390). Chicago: NSSE.

Storey, K., Bates, P., McGhee, N., and Dycus, S. (1984). Reducing the self-stimulatory behavior of a profoundly retarded female through sensory awareness training. *Am. J. Occup. Ther., 38,* 510–516.

Strupp, H. H. (1981). Clinical research, practice, and the crisis of confidence. *J. Consult. Clin. Psychol., 49,* 216–220.

Strupp, H. H., and Bergin, A. E. (1969). Some empirical and conceptual basis for coordi-

234 Evaluating Clinical Change

nated research in psychotherapy: A critical review of issues, trends, and evidence. *In. J. Psychiatry, 7,* 18–90.

Sulzer-Azaroff, B., and Mayer, C. (1977). *Applying behavior analysis procedures with children and youth.* New York: Holt, Reinhart & Winston.

Talpin, P. S., and Reid, J. B. (1973). Effects of instructional set and experimenter influence on observer reliability. *Child Dev., 44,* 547–554.

Tawney, J. W., and Gast, D. L. (1984). *Single subject research in special education.* Columbus, OH: Charles E. Merrill.

Thomas, E. J. (1979). Research and service in single-case experimentation: Conflicts and choices. *Soc. Work Res. Abstr., 15,* 49–55.

Trombly, C. A. (1982). *Occupational therapy for physical dysfunction* (2nd ed.). Baltimore: Williams & Wilkins.

Tryon, W. W. (1982). A simplified time-series analysis for evaluating treatment interventions. *J. Appl. Behav. Anal., 15,* 423–429.

Ulman, J. D., and Sulzer-Azaroff, B. (1975). Multielement baseline design in educational research. In E. Ramp and G. Semb (Eds.), *Behavior analysis: Areas of research and application.* Englewood Cliffs, NJ: Prentice-Hall.

Van Deusen, J. (1983). Normative data for ninety-three elderly persons on the Schenkenberg Line Bisection Test. *Phys. Occup. Ther. Geriatr., 3,* 49–54.

Van Houten, R. (1979). Social validation: The evaluation of standards of competency for target behavior. *J. Appl. Behav. Anal., 12,* 581–591.

Wampold, B., and Furlong, M. J. (1981). The heuristics of visual inference. *Behav. Assessment, 3,* 79–92.

Watson, P. J., and Workman, E. A. (1981). The nonconcurrent multiple baseline across individuals design: An extension of the traditional multiple baseline design. *J. Behav. Ther. Exp. Psychiatry, 12,* 257–259.

Webb, E. J., Campbell, D. T., Schwartz, R., and Sechrest, L. (1981). *Nonreactive measures in the social sciences* (2nd ed.). Boston: Houghton-Mifflin.

Weiss, C. (1972). *Evaluating action programs: Readings in social action and education.* Boston: Allyn & Bacon.

White, O. R. (1971). *Pragmatic approaches to progress in the single case. Dissertation Abstr. Int., 32(9),* 5078A(University Microfilms No. 72-8618).

White, O. R. (1972). *A manual for the calculation and use of the median slope—a technique of progress estimation and prediction in the single case.* Eugene, OR: Regional Resource Center for Handicapped Children, University of Oregon.

White, O. R. (1974). *The ''split-middle'' a ''quickie'' method of trend estimation.* Seattle: University of Washington, Experimental Education Unit, Child Development and Mental Retardation Center.

White, O. R. (1977). Data-based instruction: Evaluating educational progress. In J. D. Cone and R. P. Hawkins (Eds.), *Behavioral assessments: new directions in clinical psychology.* New York: Brunner/Mazel.

White, O. R. (1984). Selected issues in program evaluation: Arguments for the individual. In B. Keogh (Ed.), *Advances in special education: Documenting program impact* (Vol. 4). Greenwich, CT: JAI Press.

White, O. R., and Haring, N. G. (1980). *Exceptional teaching* (2nd ed.). Columbus, OH: Charles E. Merrill.

Williams, B. (1978). *A sampler on sampling.* New York: John Wiley & Sons.

Williamson, G. G. (1982). A heritage of activity: Development of theory. *Am. J. Occup. Ther., 36,* 716–722.

Wolery, M., and Billingsley, F. F. (1982). An application of Revusky's *Rn* test to slope and level changes. *Behav. Assessment, 40,* 93–103.

Wolery, M., and Harris, S. R. (1982). Interpreting results of single-subject research designs. *Phys. Ther., 62,* 445–452.

Wolf, M. M. (1978). Social validity: The case for subjective measurement, or how applied behavior analysis is finding its heart. *J. Appl. Behav. Anal., 11,* 203–214.

Yeaton, W. H. (1982). A critique of the effectiveness of applied behavior analysis research. *Advanced Behav. Res. Ther., 4,* 75–96.

Yin, R. K. (1984). *Case study research: Design and methods.* Beverly Hills, CA: Sage Publications.

Ysseldyke, J. E., Sabatino, D. A., and Lamanna, J. (1973). Convergent and discriminant validity of the Peabody Individual Achievement Test with educable mentally retarded children *Psychol. Schools, 10,* 200–204.

Author Index

Altmann, J. 71
Anderson, S. 16
Attridge, C. 66

Baer, D. 55, 119, 138, 144, 147, 152, 164, 166, 167, 168, 200
Bakan, D. 37, 39, 168, 194
Ball, S. 16
Ballin, A. 8, 59
Barlow, D. 8, 39, 48, 55, 78, 79, 82, 98, 108, 117, 122, 129, 152, 167, 205, 206, 207, 208, 209, 213, 214
Basmajian, J. 3, 215
Bayley, N. 27
Bergin, A. 40
Bijou, S. 65, 84, 86
Billingsley, F. 178
Birnbauer, J. 205, 208
Bloom, M. 44, 45, 56, 58, 78, 85, 97, 148, 152, 158, 170, 183, 185, 186, 189, 195, 204, 212
Blumberg, C. 189
Bolgar, H. 59
Bolstad, O. 84
Bonadonna, P. 69, 72
Bracht, G. 31
Brody, G. 178, 195
Bryan, A. 118
Burr, W. 8, 9

Campbell, D. 19, 24, 25, 32, 33, 53, 56, 80, 91, 166, 198, 199
Carr, B. 76
Cartwright, C. 68
Cartwright, G. 68
Carver, R. 39, 168, 194
Chassan, J. 54, 57
Chee, F. 8, 9
Christensen, L. 167

Christiansen, C. 3, 8, 31
Cohen, S. 165, 168, 194, 200
Connolly, B. 94
Cook, T. 15, 19, 24, 25, 53, 166, 199
Cooper, H. 169
Cooper, J. 79
Cox, R. 92
Cronbach, L. 15, 16, 18, 56
Cubie, S. 92
Cuvo, A. 118, 121

Denenberg, V. 206
Denny, T. 16
DeProspero, A. 165, 168, 194, 200
Dotson, V. 84
Dubois, E. 155

Edington, E. 122, 178, 193
Edwards, A. 155
Elashoff, J. 195
Epstein, S. 205

Fischer, J. 44, 45, 56, 58, 78, 85, 97, 152, 158, 170, 186, 189, 195, 204, 212
Fisher, R. 30, 148
Fishman, S. 59
Foster, D. 53
Freeman, H. 18
Fuhrer, M. 8
Furlong, M. 165, 168, 198, 200

Gast, D. 83, 98, 119, 138, 144, 147, 151, 152, 155, 157, 198
Gentile, J. 179
Gilbert, J. 169
Gillette, N. 4, 43
Girman, S. 186
Glass, G. 31, 165, 166, 170, 171, 173, 186, 193, 194, 200

Goode, W. 7
Goodisman, L. 66, 67
Gortner, S. 7
Gottman, J. 165, 166, 170, 173, 188, 193, 194, 200
Greenwald, A. 194

Hacker, B. 198
Hallahan, D. 13
Haring, N. 76, 147, 155, 157
Harris, F. 85, 148, 157
Hartmann, D. 122, 130, 169, 170, 173, 180
Hawkins, R. 67, 72, 84
Hayes, S. 103, 122, 126, 129, 162
Haynes, S. 80
Hemphill, J. 15
Herbert, J. 66
Hersen, M. 39, 48, 55, 79, 98, 108, 117, 167, 205, 206, 207, 208, 209
Hislop, H. 3
Horn, W. 80
Horner, R. 119
Huitema, B. 174, 186
Hunt, J. 8, 59

Isaac, S. 33

Jackson, D. 84
Jayaratne, S. 57, 109, 173, 174, 180, 182, 188
Johnson, S. 84
Johnston, J. 51, 67, 193
Jones, R. 165, 166, 170, 174, 200
Kaplan, K. 92
Kauffman, J. 13
Kazdin, A. 44, 51, 53, 55, 56, 79, 80, 93, 94, 108, 109, 113, 122, 130, 137, 138, 147, 156, 157, 165, 167, 168, 169, 185, 193, 195, 198, 204, 206, 209, 210, 211
Kelly, M. 84, 85
Kendall, L. 79
Keppel, G. 31
Kerlinger, F. 31
Ketefian, S. 7
Kirk, R. 33
Koorland, M. 147
Kratochwill, T. 53, 105, 131, 178, 195, 198, 203, 204

Lahey, B. 85
Laskas, C. 99
Leiblum, S. 188

Leitenberg, H. 122, 205
Levin, R. 131
Levy, R. 57, 109, 173, 174, 180, 182, 188, 198
Llorens, L. 7
Lucci, J. 94

Martin, G. 87, 147
Mash, E. 70
Mayer, C. 122
McCain, L. 178
McCleary, R. 178
McDowall, D. 171
McPherson, J. 10
Michael, W. 33, 138, 167, 168, 180, 195
Murphy, R. 118

Nahm, H. 7
Nelson, R. 97, 126
Noonan, M. 121

Olson, D. 198
Orelove, F. 67, 101
Ottenbacher, K. 1, 2, 7, 39, 95, 96, 106, 114, 122, 203, 205

Parsonson, B. 138, 144, 147, 152, 164, 166, 168, 200
Payton, O. 4, 43
Pear, J. 87
Pennypacker, H. 51, 67, 147, 193
Popham, W. 16

Ray, S. 97, 99, 203
Reichardt, C. 15
Reid, J. 80
Repp, A. 72, 73, 80
Robinson, P. 30, 53
Rosenthal, R. 29, 37
Rosnow, R. 37
Rossi, P. 18

Sackett, G. 72
Sanders, R. 144
Schenkenberg, T. 126
Short, M. 1, 2, 7
Sidman, M. 54, 132, 167, 194, 206, 207
Smith, P. 79
Sobsey, R. 67, 101
Stake, R. 16
Stanley, J. 25, 32, 33, 56, 80, 91, 198
Storey, K. 128

Strupp, H. 8, 40, 59
Sulzer-Azaroff, B. 122, 131, 132

Talpin, P. 80
Tawney, J. 83, 98, 119, 138, 144, 147, 151, 152, 155, 157, 198
Thomas, E. 99, 108
Thoreson, C. 195
Trombly, C. 10, 126
Tryon, W. 152, 178, 189, 192

Ulman, J. 131, 132

Van Deusen, J. 126
Van Houten, R. 211

Wallace, R. 84
Wampold, B. 165, 168, 198, 200
Watson, P. 116, 117
Webb, E. 51
West, W. 92
White, O. 52, 54, 59, 76, 147, 155, 157, 165, 185, 198, 203
Williams, B. 31, 76
Willamson, G. 9
Wolery, M. 148, 157, 178
Wolf, M. 79, 209, 211
Workman, E. 116, 117

Yeaton, W. 211
Yin, R. 59
York, J. 106, 114, 122
Ysseldyke, J. 79

Subject Index

AB design 46–47, 95–98, 172–174, 182–183, 201–202, 217
ABA design 98–100, 217
ABAB design 100–103, 162–163, 206, 217
Alternating treatment design 122–129, 217
Autocorrelation 171–174, 217

BAB design 103–105, 217
Bartlett's test 173–174
Baseline 74, 107–108, 218
Behavior 66–68, 218
Between-subject 56, 61, 201–202
Binomial test 185

C-statistic 152–153, 189–193
Carry over effect 129–132, 218
Case study 91–95, 218
Ceiling effect 218
Celeration line 155–160, 218
Changing criterion design 105–107, 218
Clinical replication 208–209
Clinical significance 138, 164–166, 168–170, 200
Collecting data 69–74, 108–109
Control group 24, 201–202, 218
Correlation 34, 218
Correlational design 34
Counterbalance 130–132, 219
Counterinstance 93–94
Cycling behavior 186, 198–199

Data 219
Data path 139–140, 147–148
Data point 219
Data recording form 74–75
Dependent variable 21–22, 219
Direct replication 205–207
Duration recording 71, 219

Ecological inventory 13–14
Ecological validity 31, 219
Empirical method 8–10, 219
Error 194
Evaluation 17–19, 219
Event recording 70–71
Ex post facto design 35, 220
Experimental control 90
Experimental design 32
Experimental group 24
External validity 31–32, 53–55, 204–205, 220

First difference transformation 174–177
Floor effect 220
Frequency recording 220
Functional definitions 68

Graphs
  analysis of 139–148
  bar 141–144
  cumulative 141, 219
  histogram 141–144, 220
  labeling of 148
  scaling of 145–147
  simple line 139–140, 224
Group-comparison design, limitation of 37–40, 44, 82, 220

Histogram (see Graphs)
Hypothesis 22, 35–36, 220
  null 35–36
  source of 93
  testing of 24–25

Idiographic 220–221
Independent variable 21–22, 221
Informed consent 213–215
Interaction design 132, 221

Internal validity 25–31, 49–55, 198–204, 221
  control of 30–31, 198, 204
  cycling behavior 198–199
  experimental mortality 27–28, 220
  experimental bias 29–30
  history 26, 98, 220
  instrumentation 28–29, 49, 51–52, 221
  maturation 26, 98, 221
  order and sequence interaction 203–204
  reactive interventions 203–204
  selection 29
  statistical conclusion validity 199–203
  statistical regression 27, 225
  testing 26–27, 49–51, 225
Interrater agreement 84–87, 221
Interval sampling 71–72

Lag 171
Level 148–151, 160–161, 221
Linear trend 154, 156
Logarithmic scaling 147

Mean 222
Mean lines 149–153
Measurement 222
Medical model 12–14
Molar measures 78
Molecular measures 78
Moving average transformation 177–178
Multielement design 122
Multiple baseline design 49–50, 112–117, 222
Multiple probe design 119–122, 222
Multiple schedule design 122
Multiple treatment interference 129–130

Nomothetic 222
Nonconcurrent multiple baseline design 117–119, 222
Nonreactive measure 222
Null hypothesis 35–36

Observation 66–78, 108
Observer agreement 85–87
Observer drift 87
Occurrence/nonoccurrence agreement 85–87
Operational definitions 68, 222
Order effects 129–132, 203–204, 223

Parametric statistics 180
Percentage agreement 184

Percentage correct performance 73–74, 223
Phase change 223
Point-to-point reliability 85–87
Population 23, 223
Population validity 31, 223
Practical significance 223
Pretest/posttest design 223
Probability table 183–185
Probe trials 119–120
Professional belief system 11–14
Program impact evaluation 18–19
Pure (basic) research 223

Quasi-experimental design 33, 223

Random assignment 30, 32, 198, 223
Random (sampling) selection 32, 205, 223
Rate recording 71, 224
Raw data 224
Reactive interventions 203–204
Reactive measures 80–81, 224
Recording accuracy 80–83
Recording data 75–76
Reliability 83–87
Replication 54–56, 205–209
  clinical 55, 208–209
  direct 205–207
  systematic 55, 207–208
Research 224
  and evaluation 15–16, 212–215
  and practice 7–11, 197–198, 215
  and professional development 7–8
  and theory 7–11
  applied 16
  attitude toward 3–4
  clinical 5
  need for 2–5
  pure 213
  purpose of 8
  utilization of 8–11
Reversal 103, 162–163

Sample 23, 224
Scientist-clinician 212
Self-anchored rating scale 78–80
Self-reports 78–80
Serial dependency 166, 169–174, 180, 186, 188, 192
Simultaneous treatment design 132–133, 224
Single-case study 94–95
Single system design
  characteristics 45–49, 90–91

definition 45, 224
  notation 45
Slope 159–161, 224
Social validation 209–212, 224
Splinter skill 14
Split-middle method 155–159
Stability 109
Standard behavior chart 76–77, 83, 147
Standard deviation 186–189, 225
Standard error 190–191
Statistical analysis 167–195
Statistical conclusion validity 199–204
Statistical inference (group designs) 35, 194
Statistical methods
  C-statistic 189–193
  celeration line 182–186
  two standard deviation band 186–189
Statistical significance 36–37, 168–170, 183–185, 194–195, 225
Subjective evaluation 210–211
Systematic evaluation (definition) 15
Systematic replication 207–208

Target behavior 67–68
Theoretical method 9–11
Time sampling 71–72, 225
Transformation of data 174–182, 219
Treatment 225

Treatment effect 22, 193–195
Treatment evaluation 15, 212–215, 225
Treatment group (see also Experimental group) 225
Treatment research 212–215, 225
Trend 153–159, 160–161, 182, 185, 225
Trend lines 155–159
True experiment 32, 56, 91
Two standard deviation band method 186–189
Type I error 54
Type II error 39, 165

Underlying cause 13–14

Variability 151–153, 160–161, 189, 226
Variable 226
Visual analysis 148–166, 167, 194
  reliability of 165–166, 194, 200
Visual inspection 137–138, 163–166, 226

Within-subject 56, 61, 201–202

X-axis 139, 226

Y-axis 139, 226

Z-value 191–192